Sameer Singh
Shweta Singh
Manish Dubey

Cleft lip and palate

LAP LAMBERT Academic Publishing

Impressum / Imprint

Bibliografische Information der Deutschen Nationalbibliothek: Die Deutsche Nationalbibliothek verzeichnet diese Publikation in der Deutschen Nationalbibliografie; detaillierte bibliografische Daten sind im Internet über http://dnb.d-nb.de abrufbar.
Alle in diesem Buch genannten Marken und Produktnamen unterliegen warenzeichen-, marken- oder patentrechtlichem Schutz bzw. sind Warenzeichen oder eingetragene Warenzeichen der jeweiligen Inhaber. Die Wiedergabe von Marken, Produktnamen, Gebrauchsnamen, Handelsnamen, Warenbezeichnungen u.s.w. in diesem Werk berechtigt auch ohne besondere Kennzeichnung nicht zu der Annahme, dass solche Namen im Sinne der Warenzeichen- und Markenschutzgesetzgebung als frei zu betrachten wären und daher von jedermann benutzt werden dürften.

Bibliographic information published by the Deutsche Nationalbibliothek: The Deutsche Nationalbibliothek lists this publication in the Deutsche Nationalbibliografie; detailed bibliographic data are available in the Internet at http://dnb.d-nb.de.
Any brand names and product names mentioned in this book are subject to trademark, brand or patent protection and are trademarks or registered trademarks of their respective holders. The use of brand names, product names, common names, trade names, product descriptions etc. even without a particular marking in this works is in no way to be construed to mean that such names may be regarded as unrestricted in respect of trademark and brand protection legislation and could thus be used by anyone.

Coverbild / Cover image: www.ingimage.com

Verlag / Publisher:
LAP LAMBERT Academic Publishing
ist ein Imprint der / is a trademark of
OmniScriptum GmbH & Co. KG
Heinrich-Böcking-Str. 6-8, 66121 Saarbrücken, Deutschland / Germany
Email: info@lap-publishing.com

Herstellung: siehe letzte Seite /
Printed at: see last page
ISBN: 978-3-659-62775-0

Zugl. / Approved by: Faizabad,Dr.Ram Manohar Lohia Avadh University(U.P)India,Diss,2014

ACKNOWLEDGEMENT

Gratitude, they say cannot be expressed in words but only felt. Yet I take this opportunity bestowed on me to express my sentiments towards all those who made this work possible.

I would like to express my deep sense of gratitude to my respected teacher and Guide **DR. IQBAL ALI** , BDS, MDS (Oral and Maxillofacial Surgery & Oral Medicine and Radio diagnosis), Professor and Head, Department of Oral and Maxillofacial Surgery, Career Post Graduate Institute of Dental Sciences & Hospital,Lucknow(U.P) India. I have been immensely fortunate to have him as my mentor. His dual post graduate experience has been vastly enriching, not only in enhancing my surgical skills but also getting into the details of diagnosis and treatment. Through his immense power of motivation, innovative ideas, tireless work, aim for perfection, tremendous sense of discipline and academic excellence made me bring out the best of me. His ability to work hard was my chief source of inspiration at my most difficult hours of completion of this work. I am sincerely grateful to **DR. PUNEET WADHWANI** (professor).Department of Oral and Maxillofacial Surgery, Career Post Graduate Institute of Dental Sciences & Hospital, Lucknow (U.P) India , for their helpful attitude from time to time.

At this juncture I would like to express my heartfelt thanks to my mother **SMT. REENA SINGH,** my father **DR. RAVINDRA NATH SINGH,** my elder sister **SMT.SMRITI SINGH,** my wife **DR. SHWETA SINGH** for their constant encouragement and moral support that helped me tide over occasional movements of distress.

DR.SAMEER SINGH

TABLE OF CONTENTS

INTRODUCTION

A cleft is a congenital abnormal space or gap in the upper lip, alveolus, or palate[1]. The colloquial term for this condition is hare lip[2]. The use of this term should be discouraged because it carries demeaning connotations of inferiority. The more appropriate terms are cleft lip, cleft palate, or cleft lip and palate[3].

Clefts of the lip and palate are the most common serious congenital anomalies to affect the orofacial region. Their initial appearance may be grotesque, because they are deformities that can be seen, felt, and heard, they constitute a serious affliction to those who have them. They have associated problems like anodontia and supernummary teeth and malocclusion[5].

The problem encountered in rehabilitation of patients with cleft deformities is unique. Treatment must address patient appearance, speech, hearing, mastication and deglutition[5].

HISTORY OF CLEFT LIP AND PALATE

There is an excellent historical review of the subject of cleft lip and palate by *Dorrance (1933)* and another historical review by *Rogers (1971)*. This introduction will be concerned only with establishing historical trends in the treatment of this congenital anomaly.[226]

THE AGE OF EMPIRICISM

In their approach to the problem of cleft lip and palate, surgeons through ages have attempted to correct the abnormal arrangement of the cleft lip and palatal tissues and achieve a "normal" appearance. *Boo-Chai* **(1966)** reported a case of successful closure of a cleft lip atapproximately 390 A.D. in China, although the surgeon's name is not mentioned. *Yperman* **(1295-1351)** was a Flemish surgeon who appears to have written the first fully documented description of cleft lip and its surgical repair. He closed the freshened borders of the cleft lip with a triangular needle armed with a twisted wax suture, a common method of suture at the time. Palatal deformities caused by syphilis and gunshot wounds interested *Jacques Houllier* **(cited by** *Gurlt,* **1898)**, who appears to have been the first to propose direct suture of palatal perforations. However, the failure rate was high, and he suggested that, when surgery failed, the region could be occluded with wax or a sponge. *Franco* **(1556)** wrote: " cleft lips are sometimes cleft without a cleft of the jaw or palate, sometimes the cleft is only slight, and at times the cleft is as long and as wide as the lip" *(Rogers,* **1967)**. In 1561 he wrote: "Those who have cleft palates are more difficult to cure; and they always speak through the nose. If the palate is only slightly cleft, and if it can be plugged with cotton, the patient will speak more clearly, or perhaps even as well as if there were no cleft; or better, palate of silver or lead can be applied by some means and retained there". It was also described in 1564 by *Pare*, who designated such a plate as an "obturateur". *Pare* **(1975)** was also the first to use the term "*bec-du-lievre*"

3

("harelip"). *Tagliacozzi* **(1597)** described a lip closure utilizing mattress sutures passed through all layers of the lip tissue. This was a departure from the prevailing technique of needle closure and figure-of-eight suture material reinforcement. Thus, in the sixteenth century, closure of cleft lip to improve appearance was widely practiced, and the need for closure of the cleft palate to improve speech was appreciated in more limited surgical circles. The origins of the present techniques for successful closure of the secondary cleft palate are found in the early work of *von Graefe* **and** *Roux*, who in 1816 and 1819, respectively, closed the cleft of the *soft palate* with interrupted twine sutures. In Roux's patient, a dramatic change in the patient's voice was immediately noted and described. Direct closure of the *hard palate* followed in 1826.*Dieffenbach* recommended that clefts of the hard palate could be closed by separating palatal mucosa from the bone. While he also recommended lateral relaxing osteotomies to close clefts of the secondary palate, he did not employ these until 1828. This technique is still employed in certain centers at the present time. Early closure of the soft palate to induce a narrowing of a wide cleft of the hard palate was mentioned in 1828 by *John C. Warren* of Boston. This approach to wide clefts of the hard palate was repopularized by *Schweckendiek* in 1962 and is currently the subject of much debate. *Langenbeck* in 1859 and 1861 emphasized the need to elevate the periosteum with the palatal mucosa, thus forming bilateral mucoperiosteal flaps. This flap technique is still in use in some centers today. *Veau* drew attention to the fact that palatal lengthening was not achieved by this technique, launching a full-scale attack on the technique in the Deutsche. *Zeitschrift für Chirurgie* in 1936 (Converse, 1962). He converted Langenbeck's bipedicle flaps into single pedicle flaps based on the descending palatine vessels. Modifications of Veau's basic techniques were made by *Wardill (1937), Kilner (1937), and Peet (1961),* resulting in a push-back technique for closure of clefts of the secondary palate that is widely used today. Simultaneous lengthening of the nasal surface of the velum can be accomplished by the *Cronin* modification (1957). *Mirault* introduced the modern cross-flap technique of lip closure in 1844, and since that time nearly every conceivable type of flap - triangular, rectangular, or curvilinear – has been tried. Mirault's technique remained popular and was advocated during the twentieth century by *Blair and Brown (1930)*. In1884 by *Hagedorn*,who devised a rectangular flap technique to prevent linear contracture. This procedure appears to have led to the operation of *LeMesurier* in 1949. During this period Z-plasty techniques were also used in various guises to relieve the tendency to linear scar contracture. This line of endeavor led to the Tennison (1952) low triangular flap technique and the high Z-plasty-rotation flap of Millard (1958).The evolution of the techniques of treatment for cleft lip and palate, therapy for ancillary problems such as dentoalveolar arch deformities   nasal abnormalities, maxillary hypoplasia, and speech difficulties had progressed to a point where, in modern times, teams of specialists have been for manage the total problem, grown too complicated for one or two disciplines alone.[226]

ETIOLOGY OF CLEFT LIP AND PALATE

Genetic factors undoubtedly play a role in the etiology of cleft lip and cleft palate. The geneticist can assess from a good family history the possible extent to which genetic factors are involved in the etiology of cleft lip, and cleft palate in a given proband and provide the parents through genetic counseling, with a prognosis for recurrence of the condition in future siblings and the potential for affecting offsprings arising from already affecting children. The role of a geneticist of the cleft lip and palate team is therefore, to determine, not only the role of genetic factors in the etiology of the condition but also as a counselor to potentially prevent the recurrence.

No single factor causes all the clinical observed cases of cleft lip or cleft palate. Even in the individual cases, the etiology is for the most part, the result of multiple factors because for the purpose of simplicity, thus discussion will be divided into three areas.

a.   Genetic factors

b.   Environmental factors

c.   Multi-factorial etiology

Genetic Factors

Genetic syndromes

A large number of syndromes have been described in which clefts of the lip and / or palate are described as one feature of the approximately 100 of these syndromes described by Gorlin et al[6,7] and approximately 30% are the results of a single mutant gene. The majority of these syndromes present with isolated clefts palate rather than cleft lip and it has been estimated that less than 3% of all cases of cleft lip and / or cleft palate fall in this category. The best example of single inheritance pattern associated with cleft lip is the dominantly inherited lip-pit syndrome described by *Fogh-Andreson*[8,7] *and Cervervenka et al*[11,10]. In this condition a high percentage of all children express pits on the lowers lip and cleft of the upper lip, the pits being generally expressed to a greater content than the cleft.

Candidate genes for non syndromic cleft lip and palate

Alexandre Kezende Vieira and Ieda Maria Orioli (2001)[10] reviewed the candidate genes for non syndromic cleft lip and palate. Non syndromic clefts of the upper lip with or without cleft palate (CL/P) occur in between one and two for every 1,000 live births but their frequency varies much among ethnic groups.

Linhage studies as well as association studies have been conducted for testing CL/P and CP candidate genes. The linkage refers to the positions of the loci on the chromosomes. When two loci area linked, the specific combinations of alleles in those loci are transmitted together on the same chromosome within the families. The association refers however to a statistical ratio between two characteristics, which may or may not be genetic, in the general population. The two characteristics would occur together in the same person more frequently than would be expected by chance.[10]

Loci candidates for CL/P and CP.

Loci candidates through association or linkage studies	Loci candidates through cytogenetic studies.
TGFA / OFC2 (2p 13)	MS X 1 (4p 16.1)
MS X 1 (4p 16.1)	OFC (6 p 24.3)
BCl 3/OFC 3 (19 q 13)	
RARA (17 q 21)	
TGFB2 (1q41)	
OFC1 (6 p24.3)	
Marker D4S 192 (4q)	

Understanding the complexity of CL/P and CP etiology is very important for a better interaction between the dentist and the family of the affected child. The better knowledge and molecular characterization of these genes will provide much important information that would directly affect the incidence of CL/P and CP.[10]

Environmental Etiology

Included in the category are those syndromes, which assess from factors in the environment that affect normal intra uterine development. These factors include teratogens. Syndromes in the category have no clear family history or inheritance pattern. The best examples of these syndromes are rare chromosomal aberrations such as

- D Trisomy
- E Trisomy
- XXXXY Syndrome in which cleft palate and/or cleft lip are present in high frequency. These conditions are because abnormal chromosomal duplication and/or assortment early in cell division in the developing zygote presumably as a result of effect of teratogens. All teratogenic actions operate against a background of genetic susceptibility and very few cases of cleft lip and/or cleft palate have been described in which environmental factors are the sole cause.

HolLova R et al (1994)[11,7] performed a serological observation of toxoplasmosis by using the methods of IFT, CFT and ELISA in mothers with children with orofacial clefts and found that a certain proportion of orofacial clefts may be induced by toxoplasmosis[11,7]

Malsume U et al (2000)[12,7] assessed the material risk factors in cleft lip and palate and found that a significantly more babies in the cleft group had a family history of clefts and significantly more mothers reported some sort of illness during early pregnancy. There were no differences as far as dietary preference were concerned but during early pregnancy the mothers who gave birth to babies with defects tended to drink less alcohol and less coffee.[12,7]

Shaw GM et al (1996)[13] came to the conclusion that risks associated with maternal smoking was more elevated for isolated CL/P and for isolated CP when mothers smoked greater than or equal to twenty cigarettes. Clefting risks were even greater for infants with the TGF allele. Paternal smoking was not associated with clefting among off spring of non-smoking mothers and passive smoke exposure was associated with slightly increased risk.[13]

Multifactorial etiology

Majority of the cases probably have multiple etiology involving in the interaction of multiple polygenes and multiple environmental factors, collectively termed multifactorial etiology.[13]

The characteristics of polygenic inheritance is as follows

1.   Gene segregation occurs at an indefinitely large number of genetic loci. This implies that the shape or size of a character is determined by many genes and thus the expression of that character follows continuous or meteric variations.

2.   Mutation of one or two genes for a polygenically controlled trail produce little effect on the overall manifestation of that trial. Thus each individual gene contributes to the whole but as an individual is of little significance.   The population thus has a great and reserve of genetic heterogeneity in polygenic traits which are buffered against drastic changes from isolated mutations. Alternatively mutation in monogenetic traits can cause lethal changes.[13]

3.   The phenotypic expression of a polygenic trait can be similar with a large variety of subtly different genotypes.   At some point, significant difference in the genotype will produce alterations in the phenotype.

4.   Phenotypic expression of polygenic traits is not only affected by gene alteration but also is susceptible to significant modification by the environment; polygenic traits are thus characterized by gene environment interaction.

5.   Occasionally polygenes act as a 'polygenic block' and exhibit a single gene inheritance pattern, but be expressed as many phenotypic characters. This may be the case with some of the multifaceted syndromes.

If we apply these ideas to cleft lip and cleft palate we can postulate that palatal shelf length, for example, is polygenic and is continuously variable from very long to very short in duration, say, to the width of the maxilla. With a given maxillary width, progressively shorter palatal shelves with show increased difficulty in coming to a point to contact for fusion during development and at a given threshold level, they will be too short to allow fusion and a cleft palate will result. This type of variations can also occur for maxillary width, tongue size and palatal height, cell of which are probably polygenic, and in practice it is probably that all factors contribute to give failure in palatal closure. While continuous variations in these measurement is characteristic, this type of theoretic model for genetic environment in cleft lip and cleft palate is usually referred to as quasi-continuous because the manifestation of the defect is all or none in its expression is present or absent. The differences the severity of cleft are good indications of the phenotypic expressions of continuous variation in a trait such that progressively short and shorter palatal shelves produce more severe defects.

To further complicate this concept, environmental factors effective in prenatal development also affect gene expression and the production of the defect. Thus we have a complex interaction of genes and environment and even when the optimal set of genetic factors is present in a given individual, the disorder may still not result unless "some thing" in the environment also is present. Thus a person at high genetic risk because of accumulation of deleterious polygenes will not produce the defect in the absence of an adverse environmental influence[7]

Observation explained by the Quasi continuous model

The quasi continuous model proposes that when an individual crosses the threshold for a defect the genes and environment interact to give rise to that defect. If these conditions persist, relative of an individual with the defect, since they have more genes in common, would cross the genetic threshold more frequently than non-related individuals. Thus the defect would have a higher

11

incidence in families with the defect than in otherwise normal families. If defects with multi-factorial inheritance are compared, the frequency within families increases with increase in the population incidence. For example for CL with and without CP, the population incidence is 1 in 1000 and the recurrence risk for the defect is 4%.

Decreased risk with decreasing degree of relationship

Decreased in degree of a relationship decreases the likelihood of the defect recurring. With single dominant gene defects, this drops by half for each generation. With polygenic characters with a threshold, the decrease per generation is greater and non-uniform. The drop from first degree relatives (sons, daughters, brothers, sisters) to second degree relatives (aunts, uncles, grandparents) is greater than from second degree to third degree relative (cousins). In cleft lip with or without cleft palate, the incidence in first degree relative is 40 times the population incidence and in 3rd degree relative 3 times the population incidence[7.]

Children born to parents with consanguineous marriages have also been shown to have a higher incidence of cleft lip and palate[7].

By the developmental homeostasis concept, an individual measure of antigenic buffering against environmental influences depends on the co adaptation of his genome and the gene pool as a whole[7]. The breakdown of developmental homeostasis may be provided by the inter mixing of population within a species, a consequences of general incompatibility between gene complexes co adapted with each population. It is well known that each phenotype is the result of interaction between the genotype and the environment The standard phenotype is the product of oncogenic development in the normally fluctuating internal (genetic background) and external environment deleterious mutation or extreme external conditions can consequently disrupt the steady state the organism. Increase in the fluctuating asymmetry can be an indicator of the likelihood of such disruption[7].

Twin Data

Dizygotic twins should have the same incidence of the defect as siblings, whereas monozygotic twins should have a much higher frequency. The scant data available for cleft up with or without cleft palate in twins confirm thus observation. Incidence of the defect in monozygotic twins in 400 times the population incidence. All these data does is confirm the high degree of genetic involvement in the etiology of cleft up and palate. *Magatio Natsume et al (2000)[11]* came to the conclusion that the incidence of CLP in Japanese monozygotic twins is almost the same as non twins. In CL group, there were more unilateral clefts than bio-lateral clefts. In unilateral group, occurrence on left side was more common than in right side. In CL/P bilateral clefts wise more common especially in male subjects.

Recurrence risk in families with an affected individual

If unaffected parents are recognized as having genes for a given tract by the presence of one affected individual in the family, then the chances for recurrence risk depends on the mode of inheritance, although once determined does not change for any subsequent offspring. For multi-factorial inheritance, the recurrence risk increases with one affected offspring, increase further with two affected off spring and so on. This is because with each affected child the parents can be assumed to carry more predisposing genes and more closer to the threshold. The figure for cleft lip with or without cleft palate fits this pattern and the risk after one affected child is 4% and increase after two affected children to 9%.

Sex differences

Twice as many males are born with cleft of the lip with or without cleft palate than females and possibly this indicate that males need fewer predisposing genes than females to cross the threshold. This idea is supported by the fact that affected females have more chance for affecting off spring than affected males. The sex difference for isolated cleft palate may be the reverse, thus the recurrence risk is higher for affected males in this defect.

Effect of degree of severity of the defect

The quasi contains model suggests that the individual with very severe defect have more predisposing genes than those with minor defects. Thus an individual with bilateral cleft of the lip and palate have more predisposing genes than the individuals with notching of the vermilion border of the lip and therefore has more risk for producing an affected offspring. This concept is supported by the face that recurrence risk for siblings of probands with bilateral cleft of the lip and palate is 5.7%, for unilateral cleft of the lip and palate, 4.2%, and for unilateral cleft of the lip, 2.5%. The continuous variation in degree of the defect also supports the polygenic inheritance concept.

Racial Influences

The mean incidence of CL/P in Caucasians is approximately one per 1000 population (Fraser 1970)[15,16.] A higher frequency of CL/P among Japanese infants was reported as approximately 2.1 per 1000, the incidence rate for CP was 0.00055. Blacks in the United States were noted to be at a consideration lower risk of CL/P than the Caucasians *(Alysworth 1985)*[17,16]. In a large collaboration survey of births in several university hospitals, the frequency of CL/P per 1000 births was 1.34 for whites and 0.41 for blacks.

A non syndromic cleft of the upper lip with or without a cleft palate (CL/P) occur in between one and two for every 1000 live births but through frequency varies much among ethnic groups. According to a recent review of literature, the greatest prevalence is found among American Indians (3.6 / 100 births) and progressively drops in Asians (2.1/1000 births among Japanese and 1.7/1000 births among Chinese), Caucasians (1.0/1000 births) and in African Americans (0.3 / 1000 births)[10].

In a review of epidemiological studies of different geographical regions of Europe and America, it was possible to conform that the various studies contain some common findings occurrence vary between 1.0/1000 and 1.89/1000.[10]

Chung C.S., Kau M.C. (1985) [18] found that the CL (P) high risk group consisting of Japanese, Chinese and Filipinos have smaller dimensions than Caucasians and Hawaiians in the variables (S-M, M-Ba) representing size of cranial base and the measurement of facial height (M-A, M-ANS), palatal length (ANS-PNS) and the mandibular length (Ar-Gn). This has significance in relation to the development of the oro-facial structure.[18]

Parental Age

Birth order appears to play no role in the development of either CL/P or LP. There is some evidence that the risk of producing an affected child is decreased in younger parents and increased in older parents *(Woolf 1963)*[19,16]*. Fraser and Calnan (1961)*[20,16] considered that the most important factor was the elevated parental and not the maternal age.

One other point of potential interest is the concept of 'developmental noise'. The genetic blue prints for the left and right sides of the body are presumably identical and any observed differences may be an expression of the effect of environmental factors on development or the degree of development instability. Developmental instability is often increased in individuals with a defect such that asymmetry from right to left sides of the body is increased. This has been reported in individuals with cleft for body dermatoglyphic patterns and the mesiodistal diameter for the first molars and thus suggests that the affected child may be unstable the other ways. The question of increased asymmetry may be of value in diagnosis and management of patients with a cleft[7].

This defect, because of its frequency (among the top five for congenital defects to afflict man) and because of its severe effects on the oro-facial complex is of considerable importance to dentists who form a crucial part of the multi disciplinary cleft palate team.

GENETICS BEHIND CLEFT LIP AND PALATE

Development of the head and face comprises one of the most complex events during embryonic development, coordinated by a network of transcription factors and signaling molecules together with proteins conferring cell polarity and cell–cell interactions. Disturbance of this tightly controlled cascade can result in a facial cleft where the facial primordial ultimately fail to meet and fuse or form the appropriate structures. Collectively, craniofacial abnormalities are among the most common features of all birth defects. The most frequent of these are the orofacial clefts, cleft lip and/or cleft palate (CL/P). CL/P results in complications affecting feeding, speech, hearing and psychological development. Patients will undergo multiple rounds of surgical repair starting in the first year of life and may continue until 18 or 20 years old. Frequently, extensive dental and orthodontic treatment, speech and hearing therapy may be required as well as referral for psychotherapy and genetic counseling. Occurrence estimates range between 1/300 and 1/2500 births for cleft lip with or without cleft palate (CLP) and around 1/1500 births for cleft palate alone (CP)[109]. It has been reported that CLP occurs more frequently in males, while the sex bias is reversed for CP, which is more common in females [110].Approximately 50% of CL patients also have CP, which is thought to be a secondary effect resulting from the defect in facial prominence fusion that precedes palate formation. CP occurring alone is therefore considered to be etiologically distinct from CLP. The majority of CL/P (~70%) are regarded as non-syndromic, where the clefts occur without other anomalies. The remaining syndromic cases have additional characteristic features that can be subdivided into categories of chromosomal abnormalities, recognizable Mendelian single gene syndromes, teratogenic effects and various unknown syndromes.

The high familial aggregation rates, recurrence risks and elevated concordance rates in monozygous versus dizygous twins provide evidence for a strong genetic component in CL/P[111].Despite this, familial inheritance is complex with simple

Mendelian inheritance considered uncommon. As a general model, it is thought that both genes and environmental factors, acting either independently or in combination, are responsible for facial clefting. While numerous non-genetic risk factors have been identified such as use of anti-epileptic drugs, maternal alcohol or cigarette use [112], much effort has been concentrated on identifying the genetic contribution. This has taken the form of direct analysis of candidate genes, association studies with candidate genes or loci and genome-wide scans using large collections of CL/P families. Many mouse mutants with isolated clefts have been described where the specific gene is known [113], and these too contribute to the pool of candidate genes. We can therefore confidently predict that many individual genes, acting either alone or within gene networks, will be responsible for the heterogeneous causality observed in humans. It has been predicted that CLP would best fit an oligogenic model where one or a few major genes were influenced by a small number of modifiers [111,114,116] Nevertheless, the intense efforts of current screening programmes have not revealed major risk factors for human clefting, and the identification of causative mutations has remained elusive. This general failure probably reflects a more complicated and diverse etiology than these studies suggested. It is therefore encouraging that several important risk factors have recently been identified directly from human analyses. Interestingly, this has been achieved using syndromic CL/P patients, where the additional phenotypic features have allowed patients to be subdivided into more homogeneous and readily analysable groups.

EMBRYONIC DEVELOPMENT

Development of the human face begins in the fourth week of gestation when migrating neural crest cells from the dorsal region of the anterior neural tube (cranial neural crest, CNC) combine with mesodermal cells to establish the facial primordia. The maxillary prominences enlarge and grow towards each other and the nasal prominences. During the sixth to seventh weeks, the nasal prominences merge to form the intermaxillary segment resulting in both the filtrum and primary palate. This region then fuses to the maxillary prominences, which form the lateral parts of the upper lip.[117].The secondary palate is also CNC derived and forms the palatal shelves, which grow out from the maxillary prominences. Mouse mutants with disruption in genes such as *Gli2*, *Gli3*, *Tgfβ2* and *Hoxa2*result in CL/P through disturbance to CNC migration and differentiation [118,120].

In the mouse the palatal shelves first appear at around E12.5 (approximately 6 weeks post conception in human) and rapidly grow in a vertical plane flanking the developing tongue (Fig. 1). A key stage in mouse palatogenesis occurs during E12.5–E13.5, when the shelves, consisting of rapidly proliferating mesenchymal cells, undergo a sudden elevation to bring them into horizontal apposition above the flattening tongue. Several genes have been implicated in palatal mesenchymal proliferation such as *Msx1* and *Lhx8*, where CP is seen in the respective null mice due to the palatal shelves failing to meet in the horizontal plane [121.122],As a general model, insufficient mesenchyme is believed to be the most common reason for CP in mice [113].

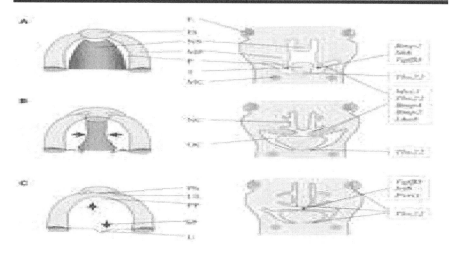

Figure 1. *Critical stages of lip and palate development. (A) Illustrations depicting paired horizontal and coronal sections of the head at mouse E12.5 (human week ~7). The medial nasal prominences merge to form the intermaxillary segment (IS) while lateral parts of the upper lip form from the maxillary prominences (MP). The palatal shelves (P) also bud from the maxillary prominences (MP) and grow vertical to the tongue (T). (B) At mouse E13.5 (human week ~8), the palatal shelves undergo epithelial remodelling and elevate to a horizontal position above the tongue. The blue arrows indicate the position of initial shelf contact and fusion. (C) By mouse E14.5 (human week ~9–10), the intermaxillary segment becomes the philtrum (Ph) of the upper lip (UL) and the primary palate (PP). The palatal shelves have fused in both anterior and posterior directions (blue arrows), together with the nasal septum. The epithelial seam disrupts and ossification begins in the anterior (hard) palate. Sites of expression for some of the key genes affecting palatogenesis are indicated in the coronal sections: yellow shading corresponds to Tbx22 expression; red indicates the palatal medial edge epithelium characterized by Tgfβ3 expression. Genes such as Pvrl1 and p63 are expressed throught the oral epithelia. E=eye; MC=Meckel's cartilage; NC=nasal cavity; OC=oral cavity; SP=soft palate; U=uvula.*

Although several theories exist for how the palatal shelves elevate, the actual mechanisms responsible are unclear. Movement from the vertical to the horizontal is likely to be a consequence of an intrinsic force resulting from increased turgidity through recruitment of water in response to elevated levels of glycosaminoglycans such as hyaluronan[123]. This occurs concomitantly with rapid remodelling of the extracellular matrix (ECM)[124]. (The shelves require the ability to hinge and maintenance of the appropriate structural shape is important during changes to the ECM and proliferating mesenchyme. *Pax9* mutant mice, for example, exhibit CP due to an abnormal morphology of the palatal shelves. The shelves are shorter and broader than the wild-type, which causes mechanical inhibition of shelf reorientation[125].Following elevation, the medial edge epithelia (MEE) of the opposing palatine shelves fuse in the midline through interactions of cell adhesion molecules and desmosomes. The palatal shelves initially contact in the mid portion and then zipper closed towards both the primary palate and the uvula. The resulting epithelial seam is rapidly removed through a combination of programmed cell death, epithelial cell migration and trans differentiation [126,127].Palatogenesis is considered to be complete in mouse by around E15.5 or 12 weeks in the human.

DEVELOPMENTAL GENE NETWORKS

A variety of molecules have been implicated in signaling facial primordial identity, epithelial differentiation and shelf remodelling .These include ECM molecules and growth factors, which act as inductive signals such as sonic hedgehog (Shh), bone morphogenetic proteins (Bmp), fibroblast growth factors (Fgf) and members of the transforming growth factor β (Tgfβ) superfamily. Shh plays an important role in the early induction of facial primordia in addition to expression in the palatal MEE[128].*Bmp2* and *Bmp4* on the other hand, are expressed more specifically within the epithelia and mesenchyme of the palatal shelves. The *Msx1*homeobox gene, which is also expressed in the facial primordia, is required for expression of *Bmp2* and *Bmp4* in the palatal mesenchyme and *Shh* in the MEE[129].Epidermal growth factor (Egf) stimulates glycosaminoglycan production within the palatal shelves while Tgfα, expressed throughout the palatal mesenchyme and epithelia, stimulates extracellular matrix biosynthesis [130].Fibronectin and collagen III act as modulating factors on hyaluronate expansion during shelf reorientation while collagen IX plays a critical role in signalling epithelial–mesenchymal interactions, appearing in the MEE cell surface just prior to shelf elevation [131].Transcription factors such as the distal-less (Dlx), Hox, Gli and T-box families also play key roles in maxillary and mandibular specification and are regulated by Shh, Bmps and Fgf signals [132].Clearly epithelial–

mesenchymal interactions are crucial in craniofacial development and specific sites of expression such as the tooth buds may function as inductive signalling centres influencing palate morphogenesis.

The TgfB family is particularly interesting in palate development and isoforms 1, 2 and 3 are all expressed during this process. Recent evidence suggests that their function in the embryonic palate is at least in part mediated through the Smad signalling system [133].*Tgfβ3* is expressed earliest and is found in the epithelial component of the vertical shelves. It is also expressed later in the horizontal shelves and MEE, but expression is undetected once the epithelial seam disrupts. *Tgfβ1* expression is limited to the horizontal shelves but like *Tgfβ3*, switches off soon after epithelial seam disruption. While TgfB1 and 2 accelerate palatal shelf fusion [134],TgfB3 may play a role in growth inhibition and is crucial for the first adhesive interaction. Indeed the *Tgfβ3* knock out mouse exhibits an isolated CP through failure of palatal shelf fusion [135,136].Although the palatal shelves otherwise develop normally, they show a marked reduction in the filopodia present on the MEE surface [137,138]and show down-regulation of condroitin sulphate proteoglycan on the apical surface of the MEE [139].Both of these are required for efficient MEE adhesion. In the mouse, antisense oligos, isoform-specific antibodies and gene knockouts show that palatal shelf fusion fails in the absence of TgfB3 but not TgfB1 or 2 [140].Tissue remodelling during palatal fusion involves a combination of basement membrane degradation and epithelio-mesenchymal transformation, both of which are under the control of specific matrix metalloproteinases (MMPs) and tissue inhibitors of metalloproteinases (TIMPs). In the *Tgfβ3$^{-/-}$* mouse, the palatal expression levels of *Timp-2*and *Mmp-13* are markedly reduced and their expression is dependent on TgfB3 [141].This model shows that proteolytic degradation of the ECM is essential for palatal fusion. Overall it is clear that tight control of a cascade of genes is required to complete normal palatogenesis.

GENETIC ANALYSIS OF CL/P

Craniofacial development is highly complex with a large array of genes implicated. Combined with multigenic inheritance and the influence of non-genetic factors, identifying the key genes in human CL/P represents a major challenge. In addition to the direct analysis of functional candidates, much effort has gone into linkage and/or candidate gene directed association studies. A major drawback lies in the analysis of patients with heterogeneous etiology, since this dilutes the chances of finding positive gene-phenotype correlations. To date four genome–wide scans for CL/P have been published, one using sib pair analysis in an English population [142], one using multiplex families of Chinese origin [143] one using multiplex families from North and South America [144] and the other using two large Syrian families[145]. The four studies do not generally concur on significant or highly suggestive regions, probably reflecting the diverse populations investigated. An exception to this is a region on 2q, which overlaps between the Chinese study and a subset of the American families. A number of new genome scans have been presented at the American Society of Human Genetics 2003 meeting, including a meta-analysis totalling 11 studies [146].Some regions consistent with previous linkage or candidate gene association studies [147] have been highlighted such as 2p13 (TGFA), 6p21.3–21.1, 17q12 (RARA), 1q22.3–41 (IRF6), and 2q35–36, as well as several new regions including, 7p13–15, 7q22-qter and 12q24-qter. It is hoped that this coordinated effort will provide the necessary power to fine map and identify the major genetic CL/P candidates.

Syndromic models for non-syndromic CL/P

Recently, positional cloning has been successful for several forms of syndromic CL/P either where rare large Mendelian families were available or where specific associated features allowed refinement of the study population. This produces a higher chance of identifying single gene causation. While these subgroups are referred to as syndromic clefts, it is now becoming apparent that the same genes contribute to the population of non-syndromic clefts, perhaps through variable penetrance or the action of different modifiers.

TBX22

We have been specifically interested in the X-linked Mendelian inherited form of CP (CPX), who exhibit a high degree of penetrance. This has been extensively studied as a rare but strongly genetic influence for nonsyndromic CP [148,157].In addition to CP or in some cases bifid or absent uvula, the majority of these patients also display ankyloglossia (tongue-tie). This minor feature is frequently missed or unreported; however, when noted in addition to X-linked inheritance, it is an important diagnostic marker for CPX. Positional cloning identified the CPX locus as the gene encoding T-BOX 22 (TBX22) [158].TBX22 is a recently described member of the T-box containing transcription factor gene family that is conserved throughout metazoan evolution. These genes play essential roles in early development and in particular mesoderm specification. The first T-box gene, Brachyury or T, was originally identified in mice [159],where heterozygous animals have short tails and homozygotes lack a notochord and mesoderm posterior to somite 7 [160]Subsequently, a family of T-box proteins have been described including 18 in humans, all characterized by a similar DNA binding domain. In addition to TBX22, several other T-box genes have been implicated in human syndromes, emphasizing their importance in development. For example, haploinsuficiency of TBX3 or TBX5 causes ulnar–mammary and Holt–Oram syndromes respectively[161,162]; TBX1 is deleted in DiGeorge syndrome[163,164];and TBX19 is mutated in isolated ACTH deficiency [165].

Although no gene deletions have yet been described for TBX22, a variety of point mutations have been identified. These include nonsense, splice site, frameshift and missense changes, with the latter affecting highly conserved residues within the T-box DNA-binding domain [166].It is interesting to note that the G118C missense mutation found in a Canadian CPX family [158,167]is at the equivalent position within the T-box domain to the G80R change seen in a Holt–Oram syndrome patient [168].This position is predicted to interact with the major groove of target DNA and has been demonstrated to result in loss of DNA binding [169,170].Taken together with the X-chromosomal localization, CP in males is likely to result from complete loss of TBX22 function, while haploinsufficient females frequently exhibit a milder phenotype.

In addition to families with clear X-linked inheritance, mutations were also found in smaller families where ankyloglossia is a diagnostic feature[158] [,171]. TBX22 expression correlates precisely with the phenotype seen in CPX patients, both in the vertical palatal shelves and the base of the tongue corresponding to the frenulum A similar expression pattern is seen in mouse[171,172]and in chick[173] The latter is interesting since birds have a constitutional cleft and one could speculate that Tbx22expression is important in palatal shelf outgrowth rather than fusion. Despite the frequent concordance of CP and ankyloglossia in CPX patients, the phenotype can vary even within single families (Fig. 2). Males usually have both CP and ankyloglossia (CPA) but occasionally CP (17%) or ankyloglossia (4%) alone. Female carriers may vary from fully affected to being phenotypically normal (CPA=11%, CP=6%, A=43%, unaffected=40%). A recent study of unselected Brazilian and North American CP patients, ascertained without bias for inheritance or ankyloglossia, showed that up to 4% resulted from TBX22 mutations[166].These include several sporadic patients with no ankyloglossia and a patient with isolated CP but with ankyloglossia only seen in the extended family. Furthermore, we have recently identified a DNA binding domain missense mutation in a five generation CP family with no evidence of ankyloglossia (unpublished data). This demonstrates that TBX22 (and therefore CPX) plays a more important role in the combined incidence of non-syndromic CP than previously expected.

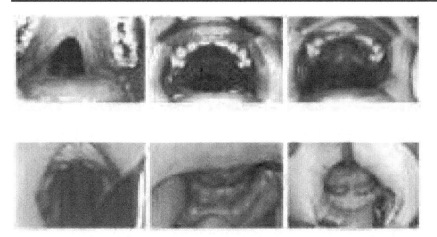

Figure 2. *X-linked CP (CPX) phenotype is variable and overlaps with non-syndromic CP. Upper panel: left picture shows the isolated cleft soft palate in the mother carrying a single base deletion (664delC) in the coding region of TBX22. The son (centre) has a less severe partial cleft but also has ankyloglossia (not shown). The daughter (right) has a similar partial cleft to her brother but is shown in the process of repair. Like the mother, she has no ankyloglossia and is a phenocopy for non-syndromic CP. Lower panel: the classic male CPX phenotype is a complete cleft of the secondary palate (left picture) and ankyloglossia (middle picture). Right picture shows the ankyloglossia in a related male with the less severe bifid uvula (not shown). His brother also carries the same mutation (TBX22IVS6+1G>C) but has ankyloglossia only with no CP (not shown).*

PVRL1

Autosomal recessive CLP with ectodermal dysplasia (CLPED1) is generally rare but occurs with a much higher frequency on Margarita Island (north of Venezuela). Positional cloning mapped the locus to 11q23 and mutations were identified in the cell adhesion molecule *PVRL1* (Nectin-1), which is expressed in the developing face and palate [174].On Margarita Island, CLPED1 is generally caused by homozygosity of the nonsense mutation W185X, while heterozygosity is high in the unaffected population. It has been speculated that, since Nectin-1 is the principle cell surface receptor for α-herpes viruses, the high frequency of heterozygotes might have resulted from relative resistance to infection by viruses such as HSV1 and HSV2[175,176]. The same mutation is also present on the Venezuelan mainland, where heterozygosity was found to be a significant risk factor for non-syndromic CLP [177].It will be important to investigate whether *PVRL1* mutations contribute to non-syndromic clefts in other geographical locations.

IRF6

Van der Woude syndrome (VWS) provides one of the best models for non-syndromic CLP since most patients have only minor additional phenotypes of lip pits and occasional hypodontia, while 15% have isolated CL/P. Linkage analysis localized the gene to 1q32–41 and mutations were identified in the interferon regulatory factor 6 gene *IRF6*[178].In the mouse, *Irf6* expression is restricted to the palatal MEE immediately prior to and during fusion. This markedly overlaps with the site of *Tgfb3*expression and may suggest a potential interaction. A common IRF6 variant (V274I) within the protein binding domain was identified in the VWS studies and has since been evaluated as a potential modifier in isolated CL/P. Transmission disequilibrium testing of >8000 individuals from 10 different populations for V274I and additional SNPs in the vicinity, shows strong evidence that *IRF6* is a modifier of CLP[179].Whilst sequence analysis in this cohort has not yet identified changes with clear causative function, a second reported study has identified an *IRF6* missense mutation in a two-generation apparently non-syndromic CLP family[180].

P63

EEC syndrome is an autosomal dominant disorder of ectrodactyly, ectodermal dysplasia and CL/P. EEC syndrome was mapped to 3q27 and heterozygous mutations were identified in the *p63* gene[181]One unusual phenomenon with p63 is that mutation to different parts of the gene can influence the cleft phenotype. Missense mutation of the conserved DNA binding domain region gives CLP while C-terminal mutations give CL or CP. Mutation at the N-terminal end outside of the conserved domains gives rise to CP or no clefting at all. Only a small number of non-syndromic CL/P patients have been screened for mutations to date and no mutations have been found[182]Not only is a larger study warranted but further investigation of downstream targets might be revealing. In particular *Jagged2*, a ligand in the notch signaling pathway, is known to act downstream of p63 and homozygous mouse knockouts of *Jagged2* exhibit CP [183]

MSX1

MSX1 first came to prominence as a candidate for CL/P following the generation of a gene knockout with cleft palate and oligodontia [121] A candidate gene-based association study reported significant linkage disequilibrium between both CLP and CP with polymorphisms in *MSX1*[184].In the same report, a cohort of non-syndromic CL/P patients were analysed for coding region mutations without success. An *MSX1* mutation was reported in a Dutch family with tooth agenesis and a mixture of CLP and CP, providing another rare example of where a single gene, and in this case single mutation, can give rise to a mixed clefting phenotype 185.Subsequently, conflicting reports have been published, some with evidence of linkage or association to either CLP or CP[186,189] and some with no association to either[190,191]. Despite these conflicts, which may arise due to variations caused by ethnic population differences, the strongest evidence for a role of *MSX1* in CL/P has now been obtained by direct sequencing. *Jezewski et al.* [192] analysed a large cohort of CL/P patients from a variety of different ethnic origins and demonstrated that up to 2% of patients, predominantly with CLP, carried *MSX1* mutations.

Other genes...

A variety of other genes causing syndromic CL/P are currently being analysed in extended cohorts as candidates for non-syndromic clefting. Examples of these include *FGFR1*, where mutations result in autosomal recessive Kallmann syndrome[193].As well as the characteristic hypogonadotropic hypogonadism and anosmia, five of the 13 patients with mutations had clefts of the lip or palate. Several forkhead genes represent good candidates, not only because of their craniofacial expression pattern but also because mutations give rise to clefts, e.g.*TTF-2* mutations cause thyroid abnormalities and CP[194], while *FOXC2*mutations lead to distichiasis, lymphoedema and cleft palate [195] .In addition, two genes have recently been identified through chromosome rearrangements in cleft patients. These are the putative transcription factor *SATB2* on 2q32–q33, which is disrupted in two unrelated patients with non-syndromic CP[196] and a novel acyl-CoA desaturase *ACOD4* on 4q21, which is disrupted in a single two-generation family with CL[197]

GENETICS[200]

The factor affecting genetics constitution resulting in   cleft lip and cleft palate deformities or both are:-

1-Mutation in genes

2-Chromosomal aberration

3-Environmental teratogen

4-Multifactorial inheritance

5-Consanguinity

6-Radiation

7-Thalidomide

8-Aminopterine

9-Diphenylhydantion

10-Trimethadione

11-Amphetamines

12-Vitamin A

13-Oligohydramnios:-Fetal Position and cortisone

14-Maternal infections

15-Alcohol in pregnancy

16-Heavy smoking at the time of pregnancy

17-Mustard gas

CHROMOSOMAL ABERRATION

The normal somatic cell contains 46 chromosomes in 23 pairs. Variation in this number is called chromosomal aberration. If an extra chromosome is present, making three chromosomes instead of usual two in particular pair, the condition is known as trisomy. There is high incidence of these anomalies in fetuses of older mothers. In trisomy 13-15 also known as fetus's syndrome, there is cleft lip and cleft palate in addition to anomalies of ears, eyes mandible and mental retardation. These infants usually die in early childhood.[201]

Multifactorial inheritance

Multifactorial denotes polygenic predisposition plus environmental insult. For cleft lip, it was noted that the ethnic difference (high in mongoloids, intermediate in whites and low in negroids) persists even after migration of these races from their native lands. This suggests that cause is mostly genetic with a relatively negligible contribution. if any, from the environmental influences[202]

Consanguinity

In many part of the World, especially in India subcontinent, cousin marriages are encouraged. In these cases deleterious rare recessive genes are more likely to meet each other; leading to disease production .Thus consanguinity is to be expected to increase the incidence of rare recessive and multifactorial disorders.[203]

Environmental factor

There is little evidence to indicate that maternal medication, minor trauma or illness play any significant role in department of facial clefts anomalies than was previously recognized. 10% of all human malformation are result of environmental factors .It is important to note that the stage of embryonic development determines the susceptibility to teratogenic development.

The embryonic period i.e. 4th to 8th week of intrauterine life, which is the stage of intensive differentiation, is more susceptible to teratogenic agent's .thus numerous malformations can occur including cleft lip and cleft palate. The effect of teratogenic factor depends on gene type and animal experiments indicate that teratogenic agent accentuates the incidence of these defects which occurs sporadically without treatment.[204]

Radiation

The teratogenic effect of X-irradiation has been known for many years and beside other well recognized defects can cause cleft palate.[205]

Thalidomide

Anti nauseates and sleeping pills is a well-known teratogen, Besides skeletal heart anomalies, it can causes cleft lip.[206]

Diphenylhydantion

This drug is used as antiepileptic in woman, has caused facial clefts beside othermalformation.[208]

Trimethadione

Another antiepileptic drug, used in past has produced characteristic congenital anomalies including cleft palate.[207]

Diazepam

It has been found responsible for oral cleft when taken in embryonic period of fetal life.[208]

Vitamin A

Johnson et al observed during their study on rat embryos, that cleft palate occurs when excessive dose of vitamin A are administered to mice in early pregnancy. They suggest that vitamin A may interfere with both early and late stages of crest cell migration during maxillary process and shelf formation.[209]

Oligohydramnios;Fetal position and cortisone

Cleft palate can result if palatal shelves are prevented from fusion by the inter- posed tongue in an abnormal fetal position[201] .In study on rat oligohydramnios was produced by treating rats with cortisone in early days of gestation. This led to lack of extension of head together with cleft palate. Corrison may have an inhibitory effect on the maturation of embryonic tissue.A Pierre Robbin's like syndrome has been produced in rats by repeated amniocentesis[211]. However the evidence that this mechanistic explanation is valid in human pregnancy is lacking. The cause for the triad of Pierre Robbin's is more likely to be genetically determined growth disturbance in maxilla and mandible leading to micrognathia and palate.[214]

Maternal infection

Certain viral diseases affecting pregnant woman in early stages of gestation may lead to congenital malformation in offspring's. Rubella virus is one of the well-known infections agent causing serious damage to the fetus. This damage results in many malformation, including central nervous system defects ,visual defects ,hearing loss ,cardiac defects ,visual defects, urogenital defect, growth retardation ,cleft lip and palate.[213]

Alcohol in pregnancy

It is occasional feature of fetal alcohol syndrome which is seen in infants born to mother who ingest alcohol in early part of pregnancy. It is occasional feature of fetal alcohol syndrome which is seen in infants born to mother who ingest alcohol in early part of pregnancy.[214]

Mustard gas

In study conducted in Tehran, it was found that chemical sulfur mustard gas was major factor in the etiology of bilateral cleft lip and palate.[210]

NON SYNDROMIC CL (P)

Development alteration predisposing to cleft lip is organized into genetic factors, environmental factors, and interactions between them.

GENETIC FACTORS:

The most extensively studied experimental animal has been the A-strain mouse. The incidence of spontaneous cleft lip varies from near zero to 25 per cent, depending on the sub line and other factors. (One observation was that some genetic effects are peculiar to the mother; i.e.. the environment she provides for the embryo predisposes the embryo to CL(P) *(Davidson and Fraser, 1986)*[25,16.] It also appears that a single major recessive gene is primarily responsible for the genetic predisposition. *Biddle and Fraser 1986*[26,16] Little evidence for such maternal effects has been found in humans. Otherwise, A-strain mice appear to be satisfactory animal models for many cases of human CL (P). Most of the facial malformations in trisomy 13 are clefts of the lip and palate.

Factors of possible relevance to this problem are racial differences in facial morphology and CL (P) susceptibility. In Oriental people there is noted underdevelopment of MNP derivatives, a high incidence of class III malocclusion (deficient maxillary components), and an incidence of cleft lip that is double that of Caucasians. At the opposite end of the spectrum are blacks, who have broad and well-developed MNP derivatives and an incidence of CL (P) that is one-half that of Caucasians and one quarter that of Orientals.[16]

In normal primary palate development there is a great deal of epithelial activity between the MNP and LNP as they approach one another. This may help to bring the prominences together and /or promote adhesion once contact is achieved. The CL/Fr strain was developed by *Fraser (1967)* by crossing A/J mice with another strain carrying a mutant gene that gave rise to a condition termed "migratory spot lesion of the retina." In offspring produced by the cross there was a higher incidence of CL (P) than in the A/J mice. Presumably the mutant gene is responsible for the fact that the epithelial activity is absent, or virtually absent, in CL/Fr embryos. It appears that the CL/Fr mouse has at least two major genes predisposing to CL(P) in this mouse. Many other abnormal genes affect primary palate development .It must be hoped that only a few will account for the genetic predisposition in most nonsyndromic CL(P) cases.[16]

ENVIRONMENTAL FACTORS:

The number of known environmental factors affecting CL(P) formation is increasing at a modest rate. Environmental factors that inhibit the electron transport chain (and consequent ATP production) are potent inducers of CL (P) in mammals and comparable clefts in the chick embryo. Electrons mostly enter the chain via the NAD-NADH dehydrogenase enzyme complex, and as they travel down the chain to progressively lower energy states, ATP is generated. Oxygen is the final acceptor of the electrons. Of the environmental factors affecting the NADH dehydrogenase complex, 6 – aminonicotinamide (6-AN) has been the most extensively studied. An interesting observation was provided by the experiments of *Landauer and Sopher (1970)*[27,16] in which they bypassed the 6-AN- induced block at the NADH dehydrogenase complex through the use of a high energy intermediate such as ascorbate (vitamin C) that donates the electrons farther down the chain beyond the block. The incidence of 6-AN- induced clefts was dramatically decreased. There is some evidence that phenytoin (Dilantin), a potent inducer of CL(P) may exert some of its teratogenic activity at the NADH dehydrogenase level.

Factors operating at the other end of the chain impeding the flow of electrons include hypoxia and carbon monoxide (CO). Although its action is complex, it appears that most of the teratogenic effect of CO is also through embryonic tissue hypoxia. The relevant human factor is cigarette smoking, which appears to double the incidence of CL(P) *(Khoury and associates, 1987)*[28,16.]

Although there have been anecdotal reports of increased CL(P) in children born to mothers living at high altitude (the 12,000 foot level, approximately equivalent to 10 percent O_2, or higher), no controlled studies have been conducted.

The pathogenesis of hypoxia-induced CL(P) has been extensively studied. The most vulnerable aspect of craniofacial development related to hypoxia appears to be the morphogenetic movements affected are the curling forward of the lateral portion of the olfactory placode, the bringing together of the MNPs in the midline (apparently mediated primarily by forebrain invagination), and the lateral flexure of the distal portion the MNP. A large amount of cell death is associated with the inhibition of lateral olfactory placodal morphogenesis owing to apparent uncoupling of the terminal web contraction.

Another CL(P) inducing environmental factor in which the pathogenesis has been studied is the anticonvulsant drug phenytoin (Dilantin). The incidence of CL(P) in the children of epileptic mothers receiving phenytoin appears to be approximately ten times that in controls. After treatment of pregnant A/J mice with phenytoin, the overall growth of the embryo, including the facial prominences, is reduces *(Sulik and associates, 1979)*[29,16] as reflected by a reduction in the fate of mesenchymal cell proliferation in facial prominences to approximately 50 percent that of controls. A finding possibly reflecting interference with oxidative metabolism reduced placodal morphogenetic movements, and /or a phenytoin-induced reduction of the epithelial activity between the facial prominences.

It was also noted that growth of the mesenchyme may normally be regulated by epithelial serotonin via the mesenchymal cell process meshwork, which presumably contains the serotonin binding protein found in that area *(Lauder, Tannir, and Sadler, 1988*[21,16]*.* The anticonvulsant, drugs are thought to function therapeutically through interference with neurotransmitters, and it is possible that at least part of their teratogenic activity may result from interference with neuro-transmitter regulation of development.[21,16]

Although not well documented, there appears to be a high incidence of CL(P) associated with prenatal ethanol (alcohol) exposure .In most cases, it is associated with fairly typical fetal alcohol syndrome (FAS), features suggesting that it may result from the same basic defect (i.e., closely set olfactory placodes and small MNPs), as suggested for trisomy [21,16]

A great deal of interest is currently being generated about the possible use of vitamins in CL(P) prevention. There is now overwhelming evidence that the recurrence rates for NTDs (neural tube defects) can be drastically reduced by such supplement. There is evidence of a much greater role for environmental factors in neural tube defects (NTD). For example, the incidence of NTDs is much higher in wet climates tan in dry climates even when the genetic background is the same. There has also been a fairly steady drop in NTDs over time, an observation that correlates with overall improvement in nutrition.

Little is known about the optimal levels of vitamins in pregnancy. There is evidence that deficiencies of key vitamins such as folic acid, which is involved in nucleotide (DNA and RNA) synthesis and thus critical for cell proliferation, can cause CL(P) experimentally. *Asling, 1961*[30,16]*:* Folate supplements alone may also reduce the incidence of NTDs in humans. *Lawrence, 1984*[31,16]*:* There is a general feeling that it is difficult to exceed an upper limit of tolerance for water-soluble vitamins (e.g., folic acid and vitamin C) in that excess amounts are easily eliminated through the kidneys. Vitamin A, a fat-soluble vitamin that is difficult to clear, may be teratogenic at high levels.[31,16]

The first major study in the use of vitamins for the prevention of cleft lip was reported by *Briggs* in 1976[32,16]. This was a multicenter study in which some pregnancies following the birth of a child with CL(P) or CP were supplemented with high levels of folate and vitamin B6 and moderately high levels of other vitamins (Stress tabs). Vitamin A was not included. The incidence of CL(P) in the supplemental group was one – third that of the non-supplemented group (borderline statistical significance.).[32,16]

SYNDROMIC CL(P)

At birth, in approximately 14 per cent of CL(P) patients, CL(P) is part of a syndrome *(Ross and Johnston, 1972)*.[33,16]

CHROMOSOMAL ANOMALIES:

CL(P) incidence is also elevated in trisomy 21 (Down's syndrome), which, like trisomy 13, involves underdevelopment of the MNP derivatives, with affected individuals resembling Orientals in facial appearance as indicated by its former name (mongolism).

In Waardenburg's Syndrome perhaps 1 percent of CL(P) patients at birth, the cleft is associated with Waardenburg's syndrome in which the incidence of CL(P) is approximately 7 per cent. The primary problem in this syndrome is abnormal development of neural crest cells. Defects include abnormalities (patchy absence) of pigmentation in the hair, iris, and skin. There are abnormalities of the inner ear (deafness in human and abnormal vestibular function in animal models).

Van der Woude's (1954) syndrome, an autosomal recessive condition, constitutes virtually the only example in which CL(P) are mixed with CPs. Lip pits are caused by abnormal salivary glands, which are often found and may be the only abnormality. Less than 1 percent of all cases of CL(P) are in this category. One suggestion concerning the pathogenesis of the development abnormality is failure of regression of the fusion epithelia.

CL(P) is also a component of many other syndromes. They provide insights into the variety of developmental abnormalities that lead to CL(P).[33,16]

NONSYNDROMIC CP

Genetic Factors:

A large tongue would be expected to interfere with shelf elevation by protruding further into the nasal cavities. A larger tongue would also push apart the midfacial halves, a finding consistent with increased facial widths in the twins. This would move the bases of the palatal shelves further apart, thereby decreasing the chances of their making contact after elevation.[34,16]

Unlike CL(P), where more than one major gene appears involved into eh etiology of most cases, an argument can be made for a single major gene in most CP patients.

Some observations regarding timing of palatal shelf elevation is made and female embryos *(Burdi and Silvey, 1969)*[34,16] may be highly relevant to the preponderance of females (4:1 over males) with CP. These investigators found that palatal shelf elevation occurs several days later in female embryos. The late elevation could put the female embryos at greater risk for even attaining shelf elevation, or otherwise would make the embryo more susceptible to other errors in position, size, or fusion that might jeopardize normal contact and fusion.[34,16]

ENVIRONMENTAL FACTORS

The secondary palate and brain are among the last structures undergoing "embryonic" stages of development (such as differentiation). Because of this, they are among the few structures sensitive to late environmental factors affecting developmental phenomena.

There is little evidence to indicate that steroids play a major role in the cause of human CP, although there have been anecdotal reports of associations between maternal cortisone therapy and births of children with CP. The possibility that stress could sufficiently raise cortisone levels to increase the incidence of CP receives little support from human studies, although interesting results have been derived from animal studies using various types of stress.

Among vitamin deficiencies known to induce CP experimentally are deficiencies of Vitamin A (retinal), riboflavin, and folic acid 1951). Excess levels of retinol also increase CP incidence.

In a study by **Khoury and associates (1987)**[28,16] maternal cigarette smoking was associated with a 2.5 times increase in the incidence of CP, which is similar to that noted for CL(P) . CPs has also been induced experimentally with fetal anoxia and hypoxia. Morphogenetic movements are also involved in secondary palate morphogenesis, a finding suggesting a possible explanation of the parallel effects concerning agents that interfere with oxidative metabolism. By this stage to development, almost all ATP is generated by oxidative metabolism, which apparently may explain the greater sensitivity of CP formation to maternal smoking.

A host of other environmental agents appear to increase the incidence of CP like phenytoin, ethanol. There is some evidence that at least part of the effect of phenytoin on secondary palate development is through interference with the steroid receptor.

GENE-ENVIRONMENT INTERACTIONS

As with CL(P), most cases of CP appear to be threshold phenomena requiring contact and fusion of embryonic primordial. For both CP and CL(P) the discordance rate of MZ twins is approximately 50 per cent, indicating that both twins are close to the threshold and that minor differences environment determine on which side of the threshold they will fall.

SYNDROMIC CP

The percentages of all CPs that are syndromic are much higher than those for CL(P)s. The variety of syndromes is also much greater.

CHROMOSOMAL ANOMALIES

CP is associated with a wide variety of chromosomal aberrations, including trisomies D, E, and G (Down syndrome).

TREACHER COLLINS SYNDROME:

This syndrome is caused by a single dominant gene .It consists of severe underdevelopment or absence of the zygomatic bone, a micrognathic mandible, external and middle ear defects, and CP in approximately 36 per cent of the cases. The clefts are wide and often involve only the soft palate region.

The following describes the apparent pathogenesis. The massive amount of placodal cell debris interferes with regional development, primarily of crest cells that become secondarily involved. The resultant underdevelopment of the proximal portions of the maxillary prominence and mandibular arch leads to malformations of the derived structures, mostly deficiencies such as those of the palatal shelves (posterior portions), which lead to CP.

PIERRE ROBIN SEQUENCE:

The syndrome consists of severe mandibular micrognathia, glossoptosis (in which the tongue blocks the airway), and variable other malformations including CP (in approximately 25 per cent), cardiac defects, and eye defects. The pathogenesis is usually considered to be decreased amniotic fluid that allows the fetal membranes to press the head down onto the chest wall and inhibit mandibular growth and movement. The resulting tongue interference with shelf elevation causes CP have been developed.

VAN DER WOUDE'S SYNDROME:

This syndrome has already been discussed in relation to CL(P). It consists of variable combinations of CL(P), CP, and lip pits (abnormal salivary glands) and is autosomally inherited, epithelial abnormality, possibly affecting breakdown and fusion, is a possibility.

KLIPPEL-FEIL SYNDROME:

In this syndrome the neck is short, with anomalous and missing cervical vertebrae. The associated CPs are thought to result from interference with mandibular, movements.

Subgroup	% Of total CP
Chromosomal anomalies	5
Klippel-Fiel Syndrome	2
Van der Woude Syndrome	1
Treacher Collins Syndrome	1
Pierre Robin Sequence	8
Total	**17**

Since this is such a late developing structure, most other craniofacial malformations have already occurred and growth distortions, therefore, could secondarily interfere with secondary palate development. In addition, clefts of the secondary palate are not life threatening during prenatal development.

SYNDROMES ASSOCIATED WITH CLEFT LIP AND PALATE[233]

1. Downssyndrome
2. Wandenburgs syndrome
3. Vander Woudes syndrome
4. Orofacial digital syndrome
5. Treacher Collins syndrome
6. Pierre robin syndrome
7. Kilppel-Feil syndrome

EMBRYOGENESIS OF LIP AND PALATE

CRANIOFACIAL DEVELOPMENT

The primary palate forms the initial separation between the developing oral and nasal cavities. It eventually gives rise to much of the upper lip, the associated dentoalveolar ridge, and that portion of the hard palate in front of the incisive foramen. It appears that almost all cases of human cleft, with or without associated cleft palate [CL (P)], are caused by failure of the medial nasal prominence or process (MNP) to make contact with the lateral nasal process (LNP) and maxillary process (MxP)

The secondary palate completes the separation between the oral and nasal cavities by forming most of the hard palate and all the soft palate. Almost all palatal clefts appear to result from the failure of the palatal shelves to make contact with each other.

ANTERIOR NEURAL PLATE DEVELOPMENT AND POSITIONING OF OLFACTORY (NASAL) PLACODES

Much of the "blueprint" for midfacial development is laid down very early (by gestational day 17 in the human embryo) at the time of anterior neural plate formation. A key element is the position of the olfactory placodes. Placodes are epithelial thickenings that play a dominant role in midfacial development. Their positioning is determined by the anterior neural plate. There is evidence that the olfactory placodes are derived directly from the anterior margin of the neural plate, separating from this margin in later development. Midline deficiencies in the anterior neural plate would consequently lead to the prospective placodes being too close to the midline. Placode positioning may be involved in CL (P) predisposition.

ORIGINS OF CRANIOFACIAL TISSUES

Neural crest cells originate from the lateral edges of the neural plate and migrate into sub-epithelial locations, either laterally under the surface epithelium or down beside the neural tube. In the head region of the human embryo, the migrations are initiated at approximately gestational day 22. As the crest cells leave the compact epithelial arrangement of the ectoderm, they adopt a loosely arranged mesenchymal appearance. Crest cells migrating beside the neural tube form primarily components of the peripheral nervous system; those migrating under the surface ectoderm in the trunk region form exclusively pigment cells, while in the head and anterior neck region they also form skeletal and connective tissues.

It is possible to produce fairly typical CL (P) s by extirpating or killing crest cells before or it the beginning of their migration, thereby reducing the facial mesenchyme and the size of the facial prominences. Consequently, the latter do not contact to form the lips and associated structures. However, this may have little or no relevance to nonsyndromic human CL (P). On the other hand, a much stronger case can be made for CL (P) s associated with Waardenburg's syndrome, which apparently involves only crest cell derivatives.

PLACODAL CONTRIBUTIONS TO SENSORY GANGLIA

Another unique feature of craniofacial development is the origin of a large number of sensory ganglionic neurons from surface ectodermal placodes. In the trunk region, all the neurons of the peripheral nervous system originate from neural crest cells.

A complicated sequences of developmental events initiated by experimentally induced cell death in the above placodal cell population at a very early age (equivalent to roughly day 27 in the human embryo) leads to, at a much later stage (roughly days 55 to 60 in the human). CP associated with a malformation complex essentially identical to the Treacher Collins syndrome. Origins and Migration of Myoblasts of Voluntary Muscles

The myoblasts that form the contractile elements of skeletal voluntary muscle originate from somites or somite like structures adjacent to the neural tube. Somites are blocks of mesoderm that form beside the neural tube, the middle layer of which forms the myoblasts of voluntary muscles. The myoblasts have a two-stage migration. The first brings the cells into the facial region as single groups related to the individual cranial nerves. During the second stage, the myoblasts migrate as smaller subgroups of cells, which may travel long distance to the final location of individual muscles. The connective tissue of the muscle is derived from local mesenchyme, almost invariably of neural crest origin.

It now appears that many, if not most; cases of CP are caused by excessive size of the tongue. The manner in which these and other muscle masses are determined is largely unknown.

DEVELOPMENT OF THE PRIMARY PALATE

At the completion of migration, crest cells surround the mesodermal cores in the visceral arches and constitute the entire facial mesenchymal cell population above the developing oral cavity. Endothelia capillary buds from the mesodermal cores and other mesoderm invade and vascularize the crest mesenchyme, which in turn forms all of the vessel wall except the endothelial lining. At this time (human gestational day 35 facial development enters a new phase with the regional growth of the facial prominence and visceral arches. High rates of proliferation in these structures may be maintained by an epithelial-mesenchymal interaction. A mesenchymal cell process meshwork (CPM) is found in close contact with the underside of the epithelial areas and the mesenchymal cells are connected by gap junctions. Both of these features may mediate the epithelial-mesenchymal interaction. This possibility has been supported by the findings of serotonin uptake by the epithelium and by the demonstration of serotonin binding protein in the underlying basement membrane that contains the CPM *(Lauder, Tannir, and Sadler, 1988)* It is known that the epithelium is necessary for the normal development of facial prominence mesenchyme in vitro and it is tempting to speculate that epithelia are involved in growth regulation mediated by serotonin via the CPM.

The maxillary prominence is formed by the proximal half of the first visceral (mandibular) arch, which bends so that its more proximal part ends up facing forward under the eye. It then grows forward at its tip *(Patterson and Minkoff, 1986)* which eventually contacts the MNP (medial nasal process). These prominences then coalesce through the phenomenon of fusion and merging.

Development of the MNP and LNP is complicated by series of morphogenetic movements. Initially, the olfactory placode sits over the corner of the forebrain, so that its media edges are more forward (ventral) than its lateral edge. A curling forward of its lateral margin initiates formation of the LNI and causes it to "grow" forward rapidly and "catch up" with the MNP, which forms at the medial edge of the placode. The curling forward of the lateral portion of the placode involves a major translocation of both epithelia and mesenchyme *(Patterson and Minkoff, 1985)* the above placodal movement and other movements involved in primary palate formation appear to be mediated by a contractile terminal web system, similar to that involved in neural tube closure.

Upon contact, the epithelia fuse to form the "epithelial seam," which undergoes partial degeneration *(Gaare and Langman, 1977)* and mesenchymal consolidation. Behind this region of fusion, spaces appear between the epithelial cells, which eventually coalesce to form the initial nasal cavity connecting to nasal pit with the primitive oral cavity (stomodeum

NORMAL DEVELOPMENT OF SECONDARY PALATE

Primary palate development has been completed and the secondary palatal shelves are beginning to form on the medial aspects of the maxillary processes. Before these stages, an inductive epithelial- mesenchymal interaction has already specified many of the later characteristics of the developing secondary palate. As the shelves grow medially, they encounter the tongue and are deflected downward .The growth of the shelves is apparently regulated by an epithelial mesenchymal interaction at the shelf edges.

When the shelves have reached a size sufficient for contact after elevation, they begin the process of reorientation. In the hard palate region they appear to hinge upward, while in the posterior region they apparently undergo a remodeling process. The shelves undergo the reorientation phenomenon if the tongue is experimentally removed.

The tongue is attached to the anterior end of the mandible and rapid mandibular growth may assist in bringing the tongue down and forward from between the shelves.

The shelf edge epithelium undergoes a sequence of developmental alterations that begin even before contact is made. Unlike the other covering epithelia that differentiate into mucus-secreting (nasal surface) and keratinizing (oral surface) epithelia, the shelf edge epithelia cease proliferation and undergo partial breakdown and other changes. The covering peridermal cells are sloughed. The underlying cells become active in the contact and adhesion through extended cell processes and the production of adhesive glycoproteins. Desmosomes form rapidly between the contacting epithelial cells to complete the adhesion.

The seam fragments, with at least some individual epithelial cells, apparently undergo transformation to connective tissue cells, principally fibroblasts. Mesenchyme consolidates the union and palatal bone formation is initiated at approximately the same time. The above sequence of changes in the epithelium goes on whether or not contact is made.

DEVELOPMENT OF CLEFT

CLEFT LIP

Various theories have been suggested to explain the development of usual cleft lip

1.   Failure of fusion between median nasal process and maxillary process (dursy- his hypothesis)

2.   Failure of mesodermal migration between the two layered epithelial membrane which results due to fusion between the two processes. The eventually leads to a breakdown and cleft formation *(Fleischmann,Veau and Stark)*.

3.   Rupture of cyst formed at the site of fusion.

CLEFT PALATE

At 7 weeks of intrauterine life two palate shelves from maxillary process lie vertically on either side of the tongue .Between 8-9 weeks of intrauterine life, tongue drops down due to growth of stomodeum and extension of the head. Thus, palate shelves become free and swing into a horizontal plane. By 12 weeks, a complete fusion of palatal shelves in midline takes place. Several mechanisms have been proposed for development of cleft palate.

1.   Alterations of intrinsic palatal shelf force.

2.   Failure of the tongue to drop down (as in Pierre Robin syndrome)

3.   Non -fusion of the shelves.

4.   Rupture of inadequate cyst formed at the site of fusion.

5.   Fusion of palatal shelves occurs one week late in females, exposing the female palate longer to teratogenic influence. Hence the incidence of cleft palate in female is greater than male.

EMBRYOGENESIS OF CLEFT LIP AND CLEFT PALATE

1. EMBRYOGENESIS OF CLEFT LIP WITH OR WITHOUT ASSOCIATED CLEFT PALATE CLEFT LIP PALATE

There are many types of clefts of the primary palate. The common (lateral) cleft lip, with or without associated cleft palate{CL (P)} may be divided into syndromic and nonsyndromic subgroups, depending on whether there are associated malformations. As will be seen below, nonsyndromic clefts may also be divided into subgroups.

2. CL (P) VARIABILITY AND ITS RELATION TO NORMAL PRIMARY AND SECONDARY PALATE DEVELOPMENT.

The authors believe that the initial contact and fusion between the MxP and MNP may be normal in many embryos that will develop CL (P),and that the critical problem is failure of the LNP to make contact with the MNP. The initial MxP-MNP fusion remains intact during the early stages of cleft formation, but in approximately 90 per cent of cases later ruptures.

Another variant may account for a number of incomplete cleft lips. The initial MxP-MNP fusion and the LNP-MNP fusion (and possibly the previous initial MxP-MNP fusion) have taken place but the MxP becomes somewhat disconnected with the MNP during its later forward growth, resulting in an incomplete cleft.

Little is known of the reason why palatal clefts are associated with some clefts and not with others. After the formation of a complete cleft of the primary palate in A/J mice, the tongue remains wedged in the cleft and presumably is responsible for the more rapid increase in maxillary width that is observed *(Simley, Vanek, and Dixon, 1971)* The increased width could in itself account for the cleft because of the failure of the palatal shelves to contact each other when they elevate, but they do not, in fact, elevate at all, presumably because of the tongue remaining wedged in the cleft. Tongue protrusion with downward deflection by an intact primary palate may be helpful for its removal from a position between the shelves.

The fact that the shelves frequently elevate in humans in the presence of complete primary palate clefts is indicated by the relatively high incidence of cleft lip without cleft palate (CL). In addition to the above specific instances, the many degrees of severity of CL (P), from lip scarring or notching to complete bilateral CL (P), indicate that the processes of contact and fusion may cease at any point.

Many different developmental alterations lead to CL (P).Normal contact and fusion of the embryonic facial prominences maybe considered to be a developmental weak point, with a wide variety of developmental weak point, with a wide variety of developmental alterations leading to its failure and CL (P). Most of the developmental alterations lead to CL (P) through failure of prominence contact.

Studies of facial morphology in monozygotic (MZ) twins discordant for CL (P) suggested that approximately two thirds of the CL (P) cases are caused by underdevelopment of the MNPs, which leads to contact failure. The twin studies indicated that many of the remaining one third of CL (P) cases result from underdevelopment of the maxillary prominences

3. EMBRYOGENESIS OF CLEFT PALATE (CP)

Major subtypes of CP are of syndromic variety. Syndromic CPs occasionally how distinctive cleft morphology (e.g., the posterior wide clefts of the Treacher Collins syndrome and the wide "horseshoe" clefts of the Pierre Robin sequence).

CPs can be produced experimentally in a variety of ways:

1.   Through interference with shelf elevation (as in corticosteroid – induced CP)

2.   Through amniotic sac puncture and interference with palatal shelf growth, either directly (as in retinal-induced CP)

3.   By earlier interference with maxillary prominence development as in retinoic acid- induced CP

4.   In dioxin-induced CP and other types of induced CP the shelves make contact and pull apart.

INCIDENCE

The overall incidence of cleft lip and palate varies from 0.5 to 3.63 per 1000 live birth. **Anderson (1942)** has studied the distribution according to the type of cleft[233].

INCIDENCE OF CLEFT LIP AND PALATE IN DIFFERENT RACES

Geographic section /Races	Incidence per 1000 live birth
Japanese	2.34
Indian	1.27
Caucasians	1.0
Negrose	0.5

INCIDENCE OF DIFFERENT TYPES OF CLEFT[233]

Types of cleft	Incidence(percent of all cleft cases)
1. Cleft lip alone	25%
2. Cleft palate alone	25%
3. Cleft lip and palate both	50%

Male predominance has been reported in combined cleft lip and palate defects and female predominance in isolated cleft palate patients. Unilateral defects are more common than bilateral defects and in unilateral defects left –sided preponderance has been recorded.[233]

PREVALENCE OF DIFFERENT TYPES OF CLEFT IN INDIA[233]

TYPE OF CLEFT PERCENTAGES

Place	Cleft lip and palate	Cleft palate	Cleft lip
Dharwad	44.3%	12.8%	42.9%
Delhi	68%	18%	14%
Chennai	84.7%	1.9%	13.3%

With an increase in parental age there is an risk of producing an affected childbirth order has significant relationship with defect. Children from a consanguineous marriage (marriage between blood relatives) show an increased incidence of clefts. Due to the increased social acceptance of cleft patients, inter related marriages(those between a normal person and person with a cleft)are on the rise. Children from, these marriages have an increased risk of having cleft defects.[233]

PREDICTED INCIDENCE OF THE DEFECT WITH AFFECTE RELATIVES[233]

Affected relatives	Predicted incidence (%)
One sibling	4.4%
Two sibling	9.0%
One sibling ,one parent	3.2%
Two sibling,one parent	15.8%

CLASSIFICATION OF CLEFT LIP AND PALATE

1. In the classification of ***Davis and Ritchie (1922)***[16,] congenital clefts were divided into 3 groups according to the position of the cleft in relation to the alveolar process.

    Group I   -   Prealveolar clefts, unilateral, median or

                    bilateral

    Group II   -.   Post alveolar clefts involving the soft palate

                    only, the soft and hard palate, or

                    submucous clefts

    Group III -   Alveolar clefts, unilateral, bilateral or

                    median

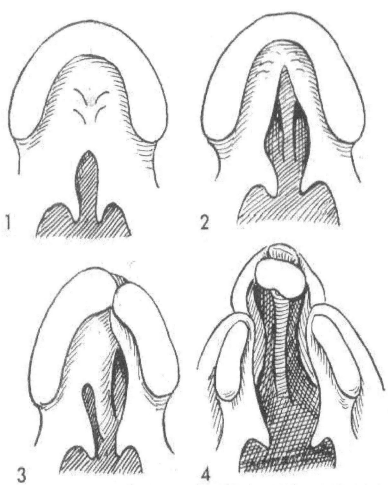

The Veau classification of the clefts of the lip and palate. Group 1: cleft of the soft palate only. Group 2: cleft of the soft and hard palate as far forward as the incisive foramen. Group 3: complete unilateral alveolar cleft, usually involving the lip. Group 4: complete bilateral alveolar cleft, usually associated with bilateral clefts of th lip.

2. **Veau (1931)**[16]suggested a classification divided into 4 groups.

    Group I   Cleft of the soft palate only.

    Group II   Clefts of the hard and soft palate extending no
    further than the incisive foramen thus involving the secondary palate
    alone.

    Group III   Complete unilateral cleft extending from the uvula
    to the incisive foramen in the midline then deviating to one side and
    usually extending through the alveolus at the position of the future
    lateral incisor tooth.

    Group IV   Complete bilateral cleft, resembling group 3 with
    two clefts extending forward from the incisive foramen through the
    alveolus. When both clefts involve the alveolus, the small anterior
    element of the palate, commonly referred to all the premaxilla,
    remains suspended from the nasal septum.

3. **Kernahan and Stark (1958)**[216,16]recognized the need for a
    classification based on embryology rather than morphology.

    The roof of the month – from the incisive foramen to its vestige, the
    incisive papilla, to the uvula – is termed as secondary palate found after the
    primary palate (premaxilla, anterior septum and lip).

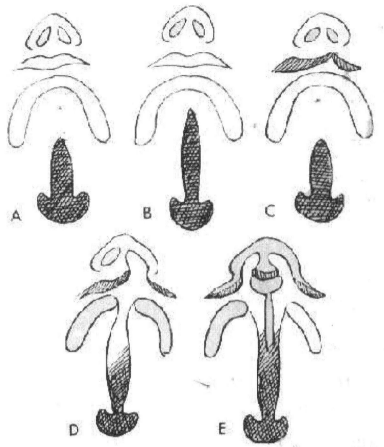

Classification of cleft palate. The division between primary palate (prolabium, premaxilla and anterior septum) and secondary palate is the incisive foramen. A, Incomplete cleft of the secondary palate. B, Complete cleft of the secondary palate (extending as far as the incisive foramen). C, Incomplete cleft of the primary and secondary palates. D, Unilateral complete cleft of the primary and secondary palates. E, Bilateral complete cleft of the primary and secondary palates. (After Kernahan and Stark, 1958.)

4.   Karnahan (1971)[16]subsequently proposed the striped Y classification

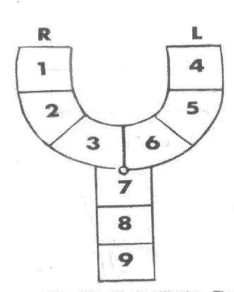

The striped Y classification. The involved
area is filled in by pen and provides graphic demonstration
of the site and extent of cleft involvement. (From Kernahan,
D. A.: The striped Y–A symbolic classification for cleft lip
and palate. Plast. Reconstr. Surg., 47:469, 1971.)

(The involved areas are filled in by pen and provides graphic demonstration of the site and extent of cleft involvement)

The incisive foramen is the dividing line between the primary and secondary palate. A cleft of the secondary palate is further classified as incomplete and complete depending on its extent.

An incomplete cleft is the common cleft of the velum, when a complete cleft involves both the velum and the hard palate as far as the incisive foramen. To this classification must be added to the cleft of the mesoderm of the palate, a submucous cleft, which may be camouflaged unless the uvula is cleft.

The incisive foramen is the reference point with stippling of the involved portions of the Y; the system provides rapid graphic presentation of the original pathological condition and lends itself to compulographic presentation.

5. **Harkine and associate (1962)**[16]presented a classification of facial clefts based on the same embryologic principles used by **Kernahan and Stark (1958)**. A modified version follows:

1. Cleft of the primary palate

    A   Cleft lip

        1.Unilateral: right, left

        (a).Extent: one third, two thirds, complete

2. Bilateral: right, left

        (a). Extent: one third, two third, complete

    3. Median

    (a).Extent: one third, two third, complete

    4.   Prolabium: small, medium, large

    5.   Congenital scar: right, left, median

        a. Extent: one third, two third, complete

    B. Cleft of alveolar process

        1. Unilateral: right, left

        a.Extent: one third, two third, complete

        2. Bilateral: right, left

a. Extent: one third, two thirds, complete

3. Median:

a.Extent: one third, two thirds, complete

1.Submocous: right, left, median

5. Absent incisor teeth.

2. Clefts of palate

A. Soft palate

1.   Posteranterior; one third, two thirds, complete

2.   Width: maximum (mm)

3.   Palatal shortness: none, slight, moderate, marked

4.   Submucous cleft

5.   a. Extent: one third, two thirds ,complete

B. Hard palate

1. Posteroanterior

a. Extent: one third, two thirds, complete

2. Width: maximum (mm)

3. Vomer attachment: right, left, absent

4. Submucous cleft

   (a). Extent: one third, two thirds, complete

3. Mandibular Process clefts

A. Lip

1.Extent: one third, two thirds, complete

B. Mandible

1.   Extent: one third, two thirds, complete

C. Lip: congenital lip sinuses

4.   Naso-ocular Cleft: extending from the narial region towards the median canthal region.

5.   Oro-ocular: Extending from the angle of the mouth towards the palpabral fissure.

Spine (1974)[16] modified and simplified the above classification as follows:

Group I: Pre-incisive foramen clefts (clefts lying anterior to the incisive foramen). Clefts of the lip with or without an alveolar cleft.

A. Unilateral

1.Right (Total when they reach the alveolar arcade or partial)

B. Bilateral

1.   Total

2.   Partial On one or both sides

C. Median

1.   Total

2.   Partial

3.

Group II: Trans incisive foramen clefts (clefts of the lip, alveolus and palate)

A. Unilateral   right

B Bilateralleft

Group III: Post incisive foramen clefts

A.Total

B.Partial

Group: IV   Rare facial cleft

Tessier (1976)[217] introduced a classification system for the most complex orbits facial clefts which have attracted the attention of the surgeon since the introduction of craniofacial surgical technique. Thus system classifies the clefts in a circumferential manner around the orbit with cranial extension. All components of the individual clefts added up to 14.[217]

CLEFT (NUMBERING) SYSTEM:

The clefts are numbered from 0-14 and follow constant line or axes, through the eyebrows or eyelid, the maxilla, the nose and the lip. The orbit is regarded as the reference mark as it is common for both the cranium and the face. Clefts that are located cephaladto the palpabral fissure are directed 'north bound' and are considered to be mainly 'cranial' in nature. The 'south bound' clefts pass caudally from the palpabral fissure to become 'facial'.

Thus, the following combinations can be clinically observed

O and 14

1 and 13

2 and 12

3 and 11

4 and 11

Although the craniofacial clefts tend to coincide with these time zones across the orbit, the vascular supply and the embryonic process do not necessarily follow the same north south pathways. Consequently, the embryopathogenesis of some of the rare craniofacial clefts are not easily explained.[217]

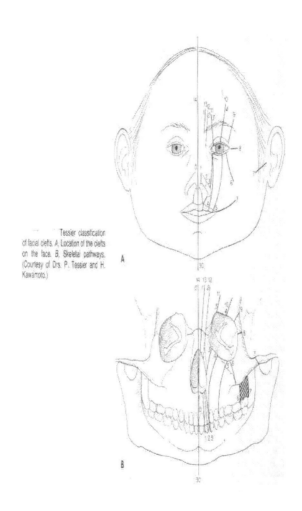

Tessier classification of facial clefts. A. Location of the clefts on the face. B. Skeletal pathways. (Courtesy of Drs. P. Tessier and H. Kawamoto.)

PROBLEMS OF THE CLEFT AFFLICTED INDIVIDUAL

A cleft of the alveolus can often affect the development of the primary and permanent teeth and the jaw itself .The most common problems may be related to congenital absence of the teeth and ,ironically, supernumerary teeth. The cleft usually extends between the lateral incisor and canine area. These teeth, because of their proximity to the cleft, may be absent: when present, they may be severally displaced, so that eruption into the cleft margin is common. These teeth usually must be removed at some point during the child's development. However ,they may be retained if they can furnished any useful function in patient's overall dental rehabilitation, frequently ,supernumerary teeth of the permanent dentition are left until 2 to 3 months before alveolar cleft bone grafting ,because these teeth ,although non-functional ,maintain the surrounding alveolar bone. If extracted earlier .this bone may resorb .making the alveolar cleft larger[218].

MALOCCLUSION

Individual affected with cleft deformities, especially those of the palate, show skeletal discrepancies between the size, shape, and position of their jaw. Class III malocclusion, seen in most cases, is caused by many factors. Retarder maxillary growth is most responsible factor for malocclusion. The operative trauma of the cleft closure and the resultant fibrosis i.e. scar contracture severely limit the amount of post natal maxillary growth and development .The maxilla may be deficient in all three planes of space, . Unilateral palatal clefts show collapse of the cleft side of the maxilla (the lesser segment) toward the centre of the palate, which produces a narrow dental arch. Bilateral palatal clefts show collapse of all three segments or may have constriction of the posterior segments and protrusion of anterior segment[218, 219].

FEEDING

Syringes with rubber extension tube connected to them. The tube is placed in the baby's mouth and small amount of solution is injected. These methods of Babies with cleft palate can swallow normally once the maternal being fed reaches the hypopharynx but have extreme difficulty producing the necessary negative pressure in their mouth to allow sucking either breast or bottle milk. When a nipple is placed in the baby mouth. He or she starts to suck just like any other new born, because the sucking and swallowing reflexes are normal .However, the musculature is undeveloped or not properly oriented to allow the sucking to be effective .This problem is early overcome through the use of especially designed nipples that are elongated and extends further into the baby's mouth. The opening should be enlarged because the suck will not be effective as in a normal baby. Other satisfactory methods are the use of eyedroppers or large feeding, while adequate for sustenance's, require more time and care. Because the child will swallow a considerable amount of air when these feeding methods are used, the child is not usually fed while recumbent, and more frequent burping is necessary[218].

EAR PROBLEMES

Children affected with a cleft of the soft palate are predisposed to middle ear infections. The reason for this is of anatomy of the soft palate musculature. The elevator veli palatine and tensor veli palatini, which are normally inserted into the same muscle on the opposite side, are left unattached when the soft palate is cleft. These muscles have their origins either directly on or near the auditory tube and allow opening of the ostium of this tube into nasopharynx when middle ear pressure are equalized by surrounding during change in atmospheric pressure. When this function is disrupted, the middle ear is essentially a closed space, without a drainage mechanism. Serous fluid may then accumulate and result in serous otitis media. Should bacteria find their way from the nasopharynx into the middle ear, an infection can develop (suppurative otitis media).To make matters worse the auditory tube in infants is at an angle that does not promote dependent drainage. With age this angulations changes and allow more dependent drainage of middle ear[220]

Chronic serous otitis media is common among children with cleft, palate and multiple myringotomies are frequently necessary. Chronic serous otitis media presents a serious threat to hearing because of chronic inflammation in the middle ear, hearing impairment are common in patient with cleft palate. The type of hearing loss experienced by the patients with cleft palate is conductive, meaning that the neural pathway to the brain continues to function normally. The defect is that sound cannot reach the auditory organ as efficiently as it should because of chronic inflammatory changes in the middle ear. However, if the problem is not corrected, permanent damage to the auditory sensory nerve (sensory neural loss) cans also result.[220]

SPEECH DIFFICULTIES

Retardation of consonant sounds (p,b,d,t,k and g) is the most common finding. Hypernasality is usual in the patient with a cleft of the soft palate and may remain after surgical correction. Dental malformation, malocclusion, and abnormal tongue placement may develop before the palate is closed and thus produce an articulation problem. Hearing problems contribute significantly to the many speech disorders common in patients with oral clefts[219].

In the normal individual speech is created by the following scheme. Air is allowed to escape from the lung, pass through the vocal cord, and enter the oral cavity .The position of the tongue, lips, lower jaw and soft palate working together in highly coordinated fashion results in the sound of speech being produced. If the vocal cords are set into vibration while the air stream is passing between, the voices is superimposed on the speech sound that results from the relationship of the oral structures. The soft palate is raised during speech production, preventing air from escaping through the nose[219].

For clear speech it is necessary for the individual to have complete control of the passage of air from the oropharynx to the nasopharynx .The hard palate provide the partition between the oral and nasal cavities. The soft palate functions as an important valve to control the distribution of escaping air between the oropharynx and nasopharynx this is called the velopharyngeal mechanism (velo means soft palate) .As the name implies, its two main components are the soft palate and pharyngeal walls. When passive the soft palate hangs downwards towards the tongue but during speech the muscles of soft palate elevate it and draw it towards the posterior pharyngeal wall, which is what happens the normal individuals soft palate when he or she is asked to say "ah". In normal speech this action takes place rapidly and with an unbelievable complexity, so that the valving mechanism can allow large amounts of air to escape into the nasopharynx or can limit the escape to none[219].

In individuals whose soft palate is cleft, the velopharyngeal mechanism cannot function because of the discontinuity of the musculatures from one side to the other. The soft palate thus cannot elevate to make contact with the pharyngeal wall. The result of this constant escape of air into the nasal cavity is hypernasal speech.

Individuals with cleft palate compensatory velopharyngeal, tongue and nasal mechanism is an attempt to produce intelligible speech .The posterior and lateral pharyngeal walls obtain great mobility and attempt to narrow the passage way between oropharynx and nasopharynx during speech .A muscular bulge of the pharyngeal wall actually develops during attempts at closure of the passage way in some individuals with cleft palate and is known as P assavants ridge or bar. Individuals with cleft palate develops compensatory tongue posture and positions during speech to help valve the air coming from the larynx into the pharyngeal area .Similarly, the superficial muscles around the nose involved in facial expression are recruited to help limit the amount of air escaping from the nasal cavity. In this instance the valving is at the other end of the nasal cavity then the velopharyngeal mechanism. However, in an uncorrected cleft of the soft palate, it is literally impossible for compensatory mechanisms to produce a satisfactory velopharyngeal mechanism. Unfortunately, in surgically corrected soft palates, velopharyngeal competence is not always achieved with one operation and secondary procedures are frequently necessary[218].

NASAL DEFORMITY

Deformity of normal nasal architecture is commonly seen in individuals with cleft lip .If the cleft extends into the floor of the nose, the alar cartilage on that side is flared, and the columella of the nose is pulled towards the no cleft side .There is also lack of underlying bony support to the base of the nose, which compounds the problems.[218]

Surgical correction of nasal deformities should usually be deferred until all clefts and associated problems have been corrected, because correction of the alveolar cleft defect and the maxillary skeletal retrusion will alter the osseous foundation of the nose .improved changes in the nasal forms will therefore result from these osseous procedures .Thus nasal revision may be the last corrective surgical procedure the cleft –afflicted individual will undergo.[218]

Nasal deformity causes defective articulation and resonation .Rhythms may also be disrupted because of the nasal leakage of air that makes speaking in phrases or sentences on a single breath of air very difficult.[218]

When there is velar insufficiency, there is no distortion of nasal sounds, *m, n, ng* because of their normal resonance .Some children display "cleft palate speech" without organic abnormality .This is sometimes the result of imitating parents with cleft palate speech.[219]

In some cases of sever nasal obstruction, the bilabial plosive *b* will be replaced by the *m*, thus making *me* become *be*. The voiced, linguoalveolar *d* will substitute for *n* making *no* became *doe*. The voiced velar *g* will be substituted for the linguoalveolar *ng*, thus *ring* might become *rig*. Hyper nasality may appear after removal of nasal obstruction. It is usually recommended that the child be seen by a speech pathologist so the child can be assisted in making an adequate adaptation to the newly opened nasal passages before he or she establishes poor speech habits[219].

INFANTILE PRESERVATION

Infantile preservation, or baby talk, is a carryover from early stages of speech development, usually characterized by the *w* substituted for the *r,* the *y* for *l,t* for *k* and *f* for *th*[219]

LALLING

Lalling is usually ascribed to sluggish tongue movement and is characterized by defective *s,z,t,d,r* and *l* sounds .Many children with mental retardation, cerebral palsy and, certain glandular diseases exhibit lalling.[219]

LISPING

The sounds usually defective in lisping are the *s,z,sh* and *zh* stigmatism is a term used for the s phoneme. Closely associated with the sibilant mentioned above are the fricative or affricates, *ch/tf/*and*/j/dz/.*Affricates have the characteristics of both a stop and a fricative. ***J.I.M TRIM*** annotated 18 different kinds of lips through use of the International Phonetics Alphabets. The following are the most usual classifications of lisp:[219]

Central, frontal, lingual, protrusion or substitution	*th* substituted for *s* or *z*
Unilateral or bilateral	"voiceless l" for *s,z,sh,zh,ch* or *zh*
Occluded	*t* or *d* for *s* or *z*:sometimes for *sh* or *zh*
Nasal (cleft palate snort)	Airstream channelled through nose instead of oral cavity

VOICE DISORDERS

Voice quality may be thought of as the " personality of the voice " this in turn , reflects the personality of the speaker .The quality may be nasal ,hoarse ,breathy, harsh, husky, gutturalor to have too much vibrato and other undesirable attributes .Likes other aspects of speech, dysphonia may be the result of organic , psychological or functional disorders .A voice that is too loud or too soft for the occasion is usually the result of personality maladjustment and is not an organic problem.[219]

The normal pitch of voice is dependent on age .If there is a physical difficulty such as malformation of the larynx, vocal folds, or other structures there will be a pitch problem .psychological pitch problem may be manifested in the pitch of adult male if he has been surrounded by female voices ,especially as a child[219].

QUALITY DISORDERS

The quality disorders most frequently noted by dentist are probably those of hyper nasality and denasality. These disorders may be caused by misplaced articulators, cleft palate, or malformations that alter the size and shape of resonating cavities. for examples , nasality may be the result of assimilation - the process of one sound influencing the other .Place assimilation often occurs ,for instance, when an a is adjacent to an a or an m . Nasalization becomes even more apparent when the "a" is between two nasal sounds a in man.[219]

RHYTHM DISORDERS (TIME)

Speech is sequential, and time and rhythm are important to good communication patterns .The rate of speech is the speed at which a person speaks .In English ,there is no standard rate for the number of syllables or words per second .The social and linguistic situations determine the rate .The sports announcer at a hockey game will , by necessity ,use a more rapid rate than the speaker in a more deliberate situation. The layman often blames slovenly speech on such qualities as rapid a rate , when the problem actually results from slovenly articulation .The speaker with a normal oral architecture may have poor speech because of too rapid rate and distinct articulation ,or he may have the reverse ,either one of which would result in communication problems.[219]

Early nonfluency is to be expected as a child "practices" his speech skills .If no attention is called to his easy repetition and hesitances, he most likely will progress to the normal rhythms of mature speech .primary stuttering may lead to secondary complications, If child becomes anxious concerning his speaking patterns. Tenseness and prolongations, in addition to tics and spasms of the vocal mechanism, cause fear and frustration. Thus, the vicious circle of secondary stuttering is initiated –the worse the speech , the greater the fear ; and the greater the fear , the worse the speech .[219]

Cluttering should not be confused with stuttering. Both are rhythm disorders, but the cluttered, as opposed to the stutterer, uses *"pell- mell"*speech ,is not aware of his problem, and does not struggle as he speaks.[219]

ANATOMY OF THE FACIAL SKELETON IN CLEFT LIP AND PALATE

Unilateral and bilateral cleft conditions showed a characteristic skeletal deformity that was consistently uniform in each cleft type, and the skeletal deformity is regarded as a product of abnormal growth subsequent to the initial embryonic failure of palate formation. Protrusion of the anterior premaxillary segment seen in the unilateral and bilateral conditions was caused by uninhibited growth of the bony part of the septal stem, consisting of the vomer and premaxillary bones. The maxillovomeral suture was regarded as having growth potential similar to that of long bone epiphyseal plates.

In man, except for a brief period in the embryo, the premaxilla does not exist as a separate entity. The term has been retained with reference to cleft lip and palate conditions because of its descriptive convenience and homology with experimental animals. In man, the term premaxilla is used to define that part of the upper jaw anterior to the incisive suture and the canine teeth. A cleft to the primary palate is usually thought to divide the premaxillary bone from that of the maxilla.

BILATERAL CLEFT LIP AND PALATE

PREMAXILLA

The complete bilateral cleft at birth shows a distinct premaxillary malformation characterized by a protrusion of the entire pre-maxillary bone with respect to the cartilaginous nasal septum and a protrusion of the tooth bearing alveolar process. The protrusive pre-maxillary bone obliterates the columellar area of the nose so that the lip attaches directly to the nasal tip. The total protrusion seen clinically is the summation of three factors; the abnormal forward position of the premaxillary basal bone; and possible underdevelopment of the maxillary segments as a whole, including some degree of anteriorly localized hypoplasia at the site of the canine tooth.

Alveolar bone supports or contains the incisor teeth, while the basal bone has a skeletal function. The basal bone articulates with cartilaginous septum superiorly and the vomer posteriorly. It is normally continuous with the body of the maxilla laterally. In normal structure the alveolar process is directly inferior to the basal bone, but in the bilateral cleft condition the alveolar bone is anterior to the basal bone in horizontal arrangement. The basal bone and the anterior nasal spine normally lie posterior to the anteroinferior point of the nasal septum, whereas the basal bone of the bilateral cleft premaxillae is anteriorly advanced and adapted around this septal point, and the anterior nasal spine ascends the anterior septal border. The contributions of the alveolar and basal protrusions to the overall premaxillary protrusion appear to the approximately equal.

The incisors are not rotated forward and upward, as might be thought, but have a relatively normal vertical orientation. They are supported by a thin protruding alveolar process, which commences at the level of the anterior nasal spine, passes forward over the developing incisor roots, inferior to the medial crura of the alar cartilages, and turns inferiorly for a short distance in relation to the labial surface of the teeth.

LIP AND COLUMELLA

The normal form of the upper lip, in particular the philtrum, philtrocolumellar angle, and Cupid's bow, is determined mainly by underlying musculature. Labial muscle fibers insert densely, into the skin lateral to the philtrum, which, not receiving such support, presents as the median philtral dimple. The inferior border of the orbicularis oris muscle inserts closely along the vermilion border and, together with the other labial muscles, appears to give rise to the tubercle, which is inferior to the philtrum. The labial musculature inserts thickly into the skin at the base of the columella and on the nostril floors, attaching this skin to the underlying bone. This anatomic arrangement is clearly a main factor in the development of the philtrocolumellar angle.

The medial part of the bilaterally cleft upper lip is conspicuously everted. This gives the erroneous impression that the premaxillary protrusion. However, it is also possible that the tethered lip induces forward growth of the alveolar process into a protrusive position. Other important factors contributing to the malformation must also be considered. The medial lip moiety contains no muscular tissue. It is therefore grossly deficient in bulk and lacks features of form normally produced by muscle. Extrinsic factors such as the tongue, mandible, and lower lip play a variable role.

The columella maybe clinically absent, but it is not anatomically absent. By definition the columella is the fleshy external termination of the septum of the nose, supported by the medial crura of the alar cartilages and covered by skin.

NASAL SEPTUM, PREMAXILLAE AND VOMER

In the bilateral cleft condition the inferior border of the cartilaginous nasal septum is reinforced by bone, which provides a stem like support for the premaxillary segment. This stem consists mainly of the vomer, its anterior part being formed by the premaxillae. The premaxillovomeral joint is located at a point approximately one third of the septal length posterior to the premaxillary alveolar process. The premaxillary segment consists of paired premaxillary bones jointed in the midline by the interpremaxillary suture, which represents the anterior third of the normal midpalatal suture. Posteriorly the premaxillary stem consists of paired processes joined by the suture and termed the infravomerine processes of the premaxillae. These overlap the single vomer, whose tapering anterior edge adapts closely to the nasal septum. The premaxillovomeral joint is, therefore, of a tongue and groove type, the vomer being the tongue and the oblique groove being formed by the infra-vomerine processes of the premaxillae.

The vomer adapts to the inferior border of the cartilaginous nasal septum and articulates posteriorly with the sphenoid bone. In cross section by vomer of prenatal specimens s "U" shaped, but after birth resorption occurs on its lateral surfaces to give a thin "V" shaped cross section with a notable edge inferiorly.

A slight swelling frequently occurs on the inferior border of the septum just posterior to the alveolar process at a position corresponding with the location of the premaxillovomer suture. The most likely reason for this is the presence of the paraseptal cartilages, bilateral finlike structures that articulate with the inferior border of the septal cartilage and diverge inferiorly in lateral relation to the vomer. The premaxillovomer stem, in the vicinity of the suture, is flanked for a short distance by the paraseptal cartilage plates. It is improbable that the premaxillovomer suture itself produces the swelling.

MAXILLARY SEGMENTS

The gum pads of the maxillary segments of the infant with bilateral cleft are covered with gingival mucosa. They are demarcated from the palatal mucosa on their medial aspect by a groove corresponding with the position of the palatal alveolar process, to which the oral epithelium has fibrous connections. The developing teeth are situated lateral to this groove; the area medial to it corresponds to the horizontal process of the maxilla and palatine bones, which are covered by the thick palatal mucosa.

The shape and size of the maxillary palatal processes occasionally show evidence of intrauterine molding by the tongue. The horizontal process of the palatine bone is deflected superiorly, suggesting that the embryonic palatal processes actually reached a horizontal orientation and that inferior pressure from the tongue then molded the processes superiorly. Despite the presence of the cleft and severed relations with the nasal septum and vomer, the growth pattern of the palatal bone appears to be unaffected in that bone resorption occurs on the nasal aspect and bone formation on the oral aspect.

The arch form of the maxillary segments generally appears normal soon after birth. However, the position of the maxillary segments is subject to intrauterine molding, particularly by the tongue, so that at birth they may be asymmetric. The tongue may have been wedged superiorly into one nasal cavity or the other, deflecting the septum a little and displacing maxillary segments considerably in a lateral direction, so as to enlarge that nasal cavity. After birth both maxillary segments tend to collapse medially.

DEVELOPMENT OF THE DEFORMITY

The premaxillary protrusion of the bilateral condition arises after original cleft formation in the embryo. The primary palate is normally formed by 35 days, and clefts would be apparent by that time. In a matter of days palatal mal-relationships would begin to show, subsequently developing rapidly to reach, at ten weeks, proportions comparable with those seen after birth.

The deformity seen in the 13-week fetus represents the failure and abnormal activity of embryonic growth mechanisms. The maxillary segments lose some of their normal forward displacement because of their isolation from the nasal septum. The premaxillary bones are held at the anteroinferior point of the nasal septum by the septopremaxillary ligament so that protrusion of the basal premaxillary bone is fully established in the 13-week fetus.

The protrusion of the basal premaxillary bone is evidently established by the age of approximately 10 weeks in utero. The dentoalveolar protrusion is a slowly progressing feature over a period of about seven months in utero and continues for some months after birth until the crowns of the primary incisor teeth reach a mature size.

CAUSES OF PREMAXILLARY PROTRUSION

The evidence indicates that the septopremaxillary ligament plays a key role. In the normal situation, premaxillary bone is kept in place by its early fusion with the maxilla to form one bone, and the developing dental arch is controlled by continuity of the mucogingival arch. The alveolar process develops inferiorly from the basal bone in relation to the developing teeth, which in turn are affixed to the gingiva by their fibrous follicles. The lip also influences dentoalveolar form.

The complete cleft condition never develops continuity of bony, gingival, or labial structure between the premaxillary and maxillary regions, so that the developing premaxillary segment is under no lateral restraint from any of these structures. Consequently, its attachment to the nasal septum by the septopremaxillary ligament becomes a dominant factor. Commencing as early as the sixth week of embryonic life, the ligament tends to shorten, drawing the premaxillary segment into the protrusive position with respect to the nasal septum and position in which it remains.

In the unaffected individual, there is differential growth between the nasal septum and the upper jaw; the cartilaginous septum slides forward relative to the bone, overshooting to the extent. The bilateral cleft premaxillae are carried forward by the growing nasal septum at an identical rate, since the ligament prevents their relative posterior movement. Septal growth stimulates equal elongation at the premaxillovomeral suture, so that the premaxillovomeral stem becomes much longer than normal. The additional protrusive growth of the alveolar process increases the deformity considerably, and by growing forward it may give the erroneous impression that the entire segment is being pushed by growth of the premaxillary stem.

The causative factors contributing to the deformity may be summarized thus; protrusion of the pre-maxillary basal bone is determined by the septopremaxillary ligament; elongation or excessive growth of the premaxillovomeral stem derives is motivation from the nasal septum; and the alveolar process becomes protrusive by growing in the direction of least resistance.

UNILATERAL CLEFT LIP AND PALATE

Unilateral cleft lip and palate consistently shows an associated skeletal deformity, of which the prominent features are lateral displacement of the noncleft maxillopremaxillary part of the upper jaw, malformations of the nose, and lateral distortion of the nasal septum.

PREMAXILLARY SEGMENT AND NASAL SEPTUM

The premaxillary segment, in frontal view, tilts upward into the cleft. The interpremaxillary suture is also rotated markedly, as seen in coronal sections, a finding that indicates that the upturning of the premaxillary segment is due to bodily rotation of the entire segment and not solely to a local alveolar deficiency. The cartilaginous nasal septum is very much bent laterally and upward with the non-cleft segment, to which it is attached in the region of the anterior nasal spine. The incisor teeth within the up tilted premaxillary segment later erupt with their crowns tilted and their occlusal plane sloping upward into the cleft. In an older patient this malocclusion indicates persistence of the original skeletal deformity present at birth.

The deviated nasal septum and displaced premaxillary region have significant implications with regard to the height of the middle third of the face. Normally the full height of the upper face is realized when the nasal septum is straight and located in the median plane. If one regards the nasal septum of the infant with unilateral cleft as being of normal size and proportions, the fact that it is bent means that it must also be shorter vertically. Thus the premaxillary segment to which it is connected suffers a decreased vertical dimension as long as the cartilaginous nasal septum remains deviated. The same observation may be made for the anteroposterior dimension when the nasal septum is considerably deviated. If straightened the nasal septum would extend further anteriorly, and a corresponding advance of the premaxillary segment would be necessary owing to the ligamentous connection between these two structures. The depressed middle third of the face occasionally seen in the 10 to 12 year old may represent a residuum of original skeletal deformity.

The nostril on the no cleft side is constricted and may be functionally occluded. The constriction results from deviation of the cartilaginous nasal septum into the floor, with the effect of raising the skin, and from the approximation of the alar base and columella. The ala nasi of the cleft side is usually stretched and flattened.

LIP AND COLUMELLA

If it were presumed that the labial muscle on the non-cleft side is normal in bulk and attachments, there would be reason to expect that part Cupid's bow and the philtral ridge on that side might be identifiable. However, the lip over the premaxillary segment is subjected to a unilateral muscle pull, which tends to retract it from the gingival pad over the incisor tooth of the cleft side, thus contributing to lip distortion. The latter finding can be attributed to the fact that the muscle band of the orbicularis oris inserts at the border of the cleft along the vermilion border, which turns superiorly at the cleft.

A columella may be identified in relation to the no cleft nostril, but on the cleft side it is merged with the stretched ala nasi. The columellar skin is more developed than in the bilateral cleft condition, but the deviated nasal septum and asymmetric alar cartilages jeopardize the prospects of normal development of a symmetric columella and adequate support for the nose.

VOMER AND PALATAL PROCESS

In the secondary palate the cleft may be unilateral or bilateral with respect to the nasal septum. When the cleft condition is bilateral, the vomer has a structure like that described above for the complete bilateral cleft lip and palate. It is symmetrically attached to the inferior border of the septal cartilage, tending to thin laterally in later infancy to develop a sharp inferior edge. In either case, since the deformity of the primary palate is similar, the middle third of the nasal septum distends into the nasal cavity corresponding to the side of the cleft lip.

In the event of unilateral union between the nasal septum and a secondary palatal process, the nasal floor thus formed is stretched laterally owing to the two factors dilating the nasal cavity. The noncleft maxilla is displaced away from the cleft, the cartilaginous septum is distended into the nasal cavity on the cleft side, and the horizontal palatal process is stretched so that the vomer is pulled into nasal floor. The suture between the vomer and the palatal processes of the maxilla is thus located in the center of the floor of the nasal cavity. The mucosa covering the oral aspect of the vomer where it contributes to the palate in this way is lined by ciliated columnar epithelium. The vomer makes a remarkable right angle junction with the cartilaginous nasal septum, which remains upright.

The intact side of the secondary palate, where the vomer is joined to the palatal process, always corresponds with the side to the intact primary palate. In the 6 to 7 week embryo, in the developmental stage at which palate formation normally takes place, the unilateral cleft of the primary palate favors secondary palate fusion on the noncleft side because the septum is bent and displaced toward that side. It antagonizes fusion on the cleft side when conditions for fusion are unfavorable because of the increased distance nasal septum and fellow palatal process.

At birth, both nasal cavities are functionally obstructed - the noncleft side anteriorly at the nostril, and the cleft side posteriorly at the conchal level.

DEVELOPMENT OF THE DEFORMITY

Two distinct phases were identified into the development of the deformity, in complete unilateral cleft of the primary palate. Deviation of the nasal septum toward the non-cleft side is of mild degree and similar in nature to that found later; however, the interpremaxillary suture is tilted toward the cleft, and there is inferior displacement of the cleft side premaxilla. At approximately 12 weeks in fetal life, the direction of rotation of the premaxillary region is reversed. The interpremaxillary suture becomes tilted toward the non-cleft side, and the premaxillary segment is rotated upward into the cleft. In the horizontal plane, lateral displacement of the premaxillary segment toward the non-cleft side is well established by the age of 8 ½ weeks. Such displacement is accompanied by bending of the anterior part of the nasal septum to the non-cleft side. Once the nasal septum becomes bent anteriorly, its middle third begins to distend into the nasal cavity on the cleft side. This is seen in specimens of 12 weeks and may occur earlier. In this manner the septal bending results in a narrowing of the nasal cavity on the cleft side and a widening of the non-cleft nasal cavity. The distention of the nasal septum also disrupts its articulation with the vomer and anteriorly, with the interpremaxillary suture. Normally the nasal septum is situated directly superior to the midpalatal suture. However, since the suture is displaced toward the non-cleft side and the septum is distended in the opposite direction, except in the vicinity of the anterior nasal spine where the septum and bone have a strong attachment, a dislocation of the septal keel away from the interpremaxillary suture occurs.

SIMONART'S BAND

It is frequently found that a cleft of the primary palate is bridged by a bar of lip tissue, referred to as Simonart's bar and band. Depending on its size, such a connection of soft tissue across a cleft may prevent the development of much of the skeletal deformity present in complete clefts. Substantial bridging bars usually pass from lip tissue to lip tissue. Narrow bridging bars may pass from the lip laterally to the alveolar mucosa medially, and this is associated with some protrusion of the premaxillary segment with mal-alignment of the alveolar arch.

Histologic examination of Simonart's band shows that it may be composed of muscle fibers and a substantial number of arterioles and nerves.

Simonart's band has been the focus of attention in the discussions of the pathogenesis of the cleft primary palate regarded.

1.   Simonart's band as the result of a healing process after breakdown had occurred.

2.   The connecting bridges was the result of only partial penetration of the epithelial wall or nasal fin, which at first separates the maxillary and front nasal processes and which is then normally penetrated b y mesoderm to establish the primary palate.

3.   *Tondury (1961)*, who suggested that Simonart's band may result from only partial formation of the epithelial wall in the first instances.

CLEFT PALATE

A cleft of the secondary palate involves both the hard palate and the soft palate from the uvular processes posteriorly to the junction with the primary palate anteriorly; the junction corresponds with the position of the incisive foramen on an intact skull. Normal fusion of the palatal processes first occurs in the anterior third at about 47 days and progresses posteriorly to complete uvular fusion by about 54 days. The variation in severity of palatal clefts reflects the anteroposterior progress of development, and the cleft invariably affects thus uvular area, which is the last to fuse. Deficiency of the bony palate varies from a midline notch in the posterior border at the normal site of the posterior nasal spine to a "V" shaped defect extending throughout the hard palate to the anterior limit of the secondary palate. At birth the uvular processes are usually shortened and distorted in an anterior direction, presumably as a result of the contraction of the musculus uvulae, which originate in part from the posterior border of the horizontal process of the palatine bone.

The tongue exercises great influences over the size and shape of the cleft palatal shelves.

ABSENCE OF MIDPALATAL SUTURE

In normal development the midpalatal suture between the horizontal processes of the maxillae is established at about 12 weeks of embryonic life; the interpremaxillary part of the midpalatal suture forms in the primary palate at about 6 ½ weeks.

Bone formation in the midpalatal suture must be seen as a response to the tendency of the maxillae to move apart secondary to forces originating elsewhere and not in the midpalatal suture. The five-week time lag between the development of bony support in the primary and secondary palates is another indications that growth of the hard palate in the midpalatal suture represents a secondary fill in process rather than a mechanism of basic importance to overall jaw growth.

Therefore, a cleft of the secondary palate does not disrupt a basic growth mechanism of the upper jaw. The main skeletal function of the secondary hard palate appears to be one of the mechanical supports for the partition between the oral and nasal cavities with regard to masticatory fusion. A second function involves bracing the molar segments against medial and lateral forces. The latter aspect becomes understandable when the continuity of the primary palate is breached by a cleft and a tendency toward maxillary collapse is observed. In such an event, an intact secondary palate counters the collapse tendency.

DENTAL DEVELOPMENT IN CLEFT LIP AND PALATE

DEVELOPMENT OF THE DECIDUOUS DENTITION

The deciduous lateral incisor in the cleft area of CLP in children is doubled in 37% of cases, and it is missing in 21% and 12% according to *Ranta*. *Bohn*[51,16]stated that the size of the lateral incisor is on the average larger than that of the contra lateral tooth on the noncleft side.*Abdulla and co-workers*[53,16]came to the opposite conclusion. Moreover, the average size of the deciduous teeth in children with CL/P is smaller than in non-cleft children

84

Only a few case reports of anomalies in the deciduous dentition outside the cleft region have been reported in children with cleft lip and palate. ***Grahnen and Granath***[54,16] reported two CL/P children with supernumerary upper lateral incisors, presumably on the non-cleft side.

Multiple small morphological disturbances have been found in the pre and postnatal deciduous dentitions of children with cleft lip and palate. Surgical trauma can cause enamel defects, especially in the maxillary incisor area.[55,16]

In noncleft children, the anomalies in the deciduous dentition are not as frequent as those in the permanent dentition. The only exceptions to this are the double formations. The following prevalence figures are derived from a study of 4,564 Danish children by ***Ravn***[56,16] agenesis 0.6%, supernumerary teeth 0.6% and double formations 0.9%. Values from a smaller Finnish material are similar to the Danish ones. Peg-shaped deciduous teeth have a prevalence of 0.005-0%.

The author is not aware of any previous studies about the timing of the emergence or formation of deciduous teeth in children with cleft lip and palate.[57,59,16] In non-cleft children the average age of emergence varies between races. A comprehensive review of studies of this field has been made by ***Lunt and Law***.[60,16] Emergence timing also has been shown to correlate with sickness and with growth in general. From a study of twins, to effect of heredity on the emergence timing has been estimated as being 78%. In emergence timing, there are no major differences between the sides of a jaw or between sexes.

In non-cleft children, there are only a few studies in which the mineralization of deciduous teeth has been investigated. Most of them are from the parental period. The formation timing of mandibular deciduous canines and molars has been studied from lateral and oblique jaw x-rays by ***Nystrom et al***.[61,16]Using intra oral occlusal films, ***Nystrom and co-workers*** also studied the rate of formation of maxillary anterior teeth. [61,16]

DEVELOPMENT OF THE PERMANENT DENTITION.

Disturbances in the permanent dentition of children with cleft lip and palate are manifold and widely studied. The permanent lateral incisor in the cleft area is more often congenitally missing than its deciduous predecessor (39% vs. 12%), according to **Ranta**.[62,16] Its size and shape are usually anomalous. Hypodontia is also prevalent generally; 10% in CL, 49% in UCLP, 68% in BCLP, and 33% in children with CP. [62,16] Its prevalence is higher in the upper than in the lower jaw[62,52,16] and on the cleft side in the upper jaw of UCL/P groups[62,52,16]. Morphological anomalies also occur throughout the dentition.[63,16] The average size of all the permanent teeth is smaller in cleft than in non-cleft individuals. In CL/P groups there is also dimensional asymmetry between contra lateral teeth in the upper jaw.[64, 65,16]

The eruption of all permanent teeth in children with cleft lip and palate is delayed compared to non-cleft children[66,16]. The mean delay in formation increases with increasing severity of the cleft from 0.3 to 0.6 years in the CL/P group during the mixed dentition period. In the CP group the average delay was 0.5 years[67,16]. The delay also increases with age in children with CP; from 0.6 years in the age group of 6-9 years to 1.1 years in the age group of 9-13 years. When hypodontia is present, the delay is more pronounced. However, the delay is similar in both sexes. [68,16]

In non-cleft children, the formation of the permanent teeth during the first years of life has been the subject of only a few studies, mainly of the mandibular molars. Only the study of **Nystrom et al**[61,16] includes information about the anterior maxillary teeth obtained from healthy, living children.

CORRELATIONS IN TOOTH DEVELOPMENT

The formation timing, as well as the emergence timing and the size of teeth, are linked to each other within and between the two dentitions. *Garn and co-worker*[69,16] studied the formational interrelationship of the permanent dentition over a period of 13 years. The means correlation for tooth formation was 0.4, indicating a moderate degree of relationship. Predictability between two formational events having 1 year's distance was 0.6, and it decreased to 0.2 between events having 13 years distance. Adjacent teeth exhibit systematically higher correlations information than do more remote teeth *(Garn et al).*[69,16] The term "distance gradient" describes this characteristic, which is also true for emergence timing in both deciduous and permanent dentitions. Whether distance gradient exists prenatally is not clear. The correlations between the emergence ages of corresponding teeth in the deciduous and permanent dentition vary from 0.4 to 0.9.[73,74,16]

ASSOCIATION BETWEEN TOOTH DEVELOPMENT AND PRENATAL FACTORS

There are some studies of the associations between tooth development in children with cleft lip and palate and prenatal factors i.e. factors other than postnatal-hereditary, maternal, and gestational). A positive family history of clefts has no effect on the timing of the permanent tooth formation or on the prevalence of hypodontia in the permanent dentition. However, in cleft subjects with a positive family history of clefts, the asymmetry of crown size between contra lateral teeth is more prominent than in the cases of sporadic cleft subjects[65,16]. In non-cleft children, low birth weight has been shown to correlate with delayed emergence of deciduous teeth[78,16], with delayed eruption and formation of permanent teeth[76,77,16] and with diminished deciduous and permanent crown diameters. Early position in the birth order and low maternal age also promote delayed permanent tooth formation[76,16]. Maternal diabetes and hypothyroidism are linked with larger crown sizes. Late eruption of the first deciduous tooth is weakly linked to low maternal age according to *Nystrom*[78], whereas a clear correlation in the opposite direction exists between these factors according to *Weyers*[80,16.] Short gestation is also correlated with delay in the eruption of the first deciduous tooth. However, when the age of the first tooth is calculated from conception, there is no difference in relation to the gestation length.[81]

The purpose of the study of dental development in children with clefts was to investigate the dental development in children with clefts of the lip, palate or both during the first 3 years of life. Data were obtained from children treated at the cleft Center of the Department of Surgery, Helsinki University Central Hospital, and they are comparedto previous studies of children with clefts, as well as to studies of noncleft children.[16]

Anomalies in the deciduous teeth, excluding the cleft site lateral incisor, were studied from x-rays 64 children selected from patient files. They had 97 anomalous deciduous teeth; 47 in the upper and 50 in the lower jaw. The prevalence of congenitally missing, fused, and peg shaped teeth was four times the number found in non-cleft children, which was not the case for supernumerary and geminated teeth. The permanent tooth succeeding the anomalous deciduous tooth also was usually affected. Most often it was congenitally missing. Moreover, deciduous tooth multi-anomalies were strongly reflected as hypodontia in the permanent dentition.[16]

The emergence ages of the deciduous teeth in children with cleft lip and palate were calculated form plaster casts of 473 subjects. The cross sectional material was analyzed by probit transformation. The emergence ages of the central incisors were obtained partially from a questionnaire study of 76 newborns, whose parent were asked to write down the eruption dates of the two first teeth in both jaws. No directional differences could be observed between the emergence ages of the incisors in children with or without cleft lip and palate. However, a trend toward delayed emergence was found in the canines and second molars of children with clefts. Moreover, a clear asymmetry was found in the upper jaw of unilateral cleft groups, indicating the delay of cleft side teeth.[16]

The formation of the deciduous and permanent maxillary incisors and canines was studies in 361 children with cleft lip and palate. All together, 704 occlusal x-rays of children aged from 2 weeks to 41 months were assessed, using a 13-stage scale. The early timing of tooth formation in both dentitions was similar to the reported for noncleft children. However, developmental asymmetry was noted between contra lateral. In the unilateral cleft lip and palate group, every tenth cleft side deciduous central incisors, deciduous canine, and permanent central incisor was delayed when compared to the corresponding contra lateral tooth[16]

For the formation timing, the correlations between the anterior maxillary deciduous and their corresponding permanent teeth, as well as that between the same teeth in both dentitions were studied, using the above-mentioned 704 occlusal x-rays. Only tooth pairs in which formation of the deciduous and corresponding permanent tooth had begun but was not complete were selected. Every tooth selected was compared to the tooth and stage specific mean ages of the total material. The difference was calculated by standard deviations (SD) units, and the correlation matrices were computed based on those SD units. The correlation was stronger within both dentitions than between them during their simultaneous mineralization. The relationship was of the same magnitude as those obtained from similar comparisons in earlier studies of tooth formation and emergence timing, as well as of tooth size, in non-cleft children. The developmental asymmetry in the maxillary teeth of children with unilateral cleft lip and palate also was reflected in the correlations between the deciduous and the permanent central incisors.[16]

The relationships between the emergence timing of the first deciduous tooth and prenatal factors (birth weight, length of gestation, mother's use of drugs pregnancy, birth order, maternal age, place of birth, associated anomalies, and anomalies in relatives) were assessed, as well as the relationship between the formation of the deciduous and permanent maxillary central incisors and the same prenatal factors. The correlations were, however, mostly not significant[16.]

Finally, hypothetical possibilities of a common etiology of dental disturbances and cleft malformations were discussed. This study showed that the prevalence of deciduous tooth anomalies in which tooth development is deficient were increased in children with cleft lip and palate. Quantitative deficiency in facial mesenchymal tissue is perhaps one possible cause of the cleft and may also explain the production of the simultaneous tooth anomaly. An explanation for the delayed tooth formation in cleft individuals may lie in the growth retardation of facial processes or palatal shelves, which may also be the cause of the cleft itself. A third possible connection between the cleft and the dental disturbances may be that both are symptoms of a generalized embryonal disturbance. These possible pathogenetic mechanisms are not mutually exclusive.[16]

HISTORY OF CLEFT LIP REPAIR

The surgical correction of the cleft lip deformity has a long history spanning several centuries and consists of hundreds of techniques described by different surgeons. There are many excellent historic reviews on cleft lip and palate surgery, important among them being the ones by **Dorrance (1933), Rogers (1971) and Millard (1976)**.**Boo-Chai**[227]in 1966 reported a case of successful closure of cleft lip in approximately 390 AD in China, although the name of the surgeon is not mentioned. In Europe, many techniques were used during the early Christian era. **Yperman (1295-1351)**[227] closed the freshened borders of the cleft lip with a triangular needle armed with a twisted wax suture. **Ambroise Paré**[227]in 1564 used a long needle through both lip elements wrapped with a thread in a figure-of-eight. A similar technique was being used even in the 19th century **(Pancoast-1844)**.**Ross (1891) and Thompson (1912)**[227,228,229]described angled incisions of the short cleft edges to obtain length with closure. **Mirault (1844)**[227]had described a lateral inferior triangular flap, to be approximated to a medial paring. **Blair (1930)**[227] modified this approach, and **Brown (1945)**[227]reduced the size of the triangular flap. This method was popular through 1930s and 1940s. In 1949, **Le Mesurier** demonstrated a modification of the **Hagedorn technique** (originally described in 1892), in which a quadrilateral flap is introduced into the releasing incision to create and artificial Cupid's bow.[227]

Tennison in 1952 designed a Z-plasty technique, which preserves the Cupid's bow. Though he called it a 'stencil method', it came to be known as the **Tennison** triangular flap technique.[227,228,230] In 1959, **Randall** modified the **Tennison** method by reducing the size of the inferior triangular flap, and defined the precise mathematics of the method.In 1955[230], **Millard**[227,231]described the concept of 'rotation-advancement', in which a lateral flap is advanced into the upper portion of the lip, combined with a downward rotation of the medial segment. **Skoog** (1969)[227], unable to obtain sufficient rotation, used an additional flap to balance the Cupid's bow. *Delaire*,[227,232] a French surgeon, in a series of papers between 1971 and 1986, demonstrated what is called a 'functional closure' of cleft lip, in which the nasolabial muscular orientation is reconstructed without any form of flap procedure. The concept of differential reconstruction of the orbicularis oris muscle in unilateral cleft lip repair was emphasised by *Muller* in 1989.[227]

UNILATERAL CLEFT LIP REPAIR

PRE-OPERATIVE FEEDING

Infants with unilateral cleft lip alone seldom present with feeding problems. But those with cleft lip and palate or isolated cleft palate need special attention if they are to be adequately nourished. In order to minimise nasal regurgitation and the risk of aspiration, it is advised to hold the child at an angle of 45-60° to the horizontal during feeding. The simplest feeder is a soft, frequently boiled rubber nipple with a slightly enlarged hole. For a child with severe feeding problem, a bulb syringe with a rubber catheteric tip may be required.[227]

Care must be taken not to flood the pharynx and thereby provoke aspiration. It should be noted that an infant with a major cleft tends to swallow more amounts of air while feeding, and hence he/she must be fed more frequently than a normal child.[227]

TIMING OF THE OPERATION

The selection of appropriate timing for surgical repair of cleft lip varies between surgeons. In some centers, infants are operated upon under local anesthesia in the first 48 hours of life.

Most surgeons delay lip repair until 10 weeks after birth. At this time, the lip structures would have increased in size providing the surgeon with larger tissues upon which to work, and there is ample time for complete evaluation of the general condition of the patient. Another important factor is that the parents who have lived with an untreated cleft patient for ten weeks are better prepared to appreciate the result that the cleft repair and rehabilitation present.[227]

An old tradition called 'the rule of tens' states that cleft lip surgery should be delayed until the child is 10 pounds heavy, has a haemoglobin level of 10 gm% and a WBC count of 10,000/mm³ and is at least 10 weeks old.[227]

ANAESTHESIA, POSITIONING AND MARKING OF THE PATIENT

General endotracheal anesthesia is used for all stages of lip repair. The infant is placed in folded towels with the neck slightly extended. Then the oro-tracheal tube is carefully taped into the Centre of the lower lip so as not to produce any lateral distortion. The exact points of future approximation of opposite muco-cutaneous junctions are stabbed with a needle dipped in Bonney's blue. After markings, 0.5% lignocaine with 1:2,00,000 epinephrine is injected into the lip tissue. A pharyngeal pack is not usually necessary.[227]

SELECTION OF TECHNIQUE

The goal of all techniques of repair is a normal looking lip and a normal looking nose, which will not be distorted by the effects of ageing and growth.

Steffenson (1953)[227] has listed five criteria for a satisfactory lip repair.

    1.   Accurate skin, muscle and mucous membrane union with adequate lip lengthening,

    2.   Symmetrical nostril floor,

    3.   Symmetrical vermilion border,

    4.   Slight eversion of the lip and

    5.   A minimal of scar which by contraction will not interfere with the accomplishments of the other stated requirements.

Two additional criteria were added later by *Musgrave (1971)*[227]

    1.   Preservation of the cupid's bow,

    2.   Production of symmetrical nostrils.

It has been argued that one should not compromise the chances of long-term good results by being overzealous with nostril and alar cartilage surgery in infancy.

In time, many surgeons develop a preference for a particular technique of repair. This can lead to a rigidity of thought in which all lip defects are made to fit a favourite operation without concern that another operation might better fix a particular lip defect. As a general rule, the method of lip repair should be selected which discards an absolute minimum of tissue. A strong plea should be made for the preservation of the cupid's bow.

The basic principles involved in lip repair are

a)   Rotation of the cupid's bow to the horizontal plane

b)   Restoration of lip length

c)   Muscle repair

d)   Restoration of nasal symmetry and prominence[22]

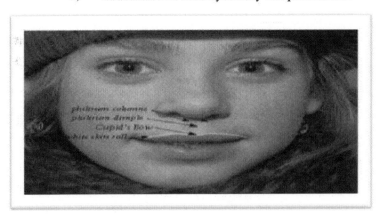

Fig.4Anatomy of normal lip[225]

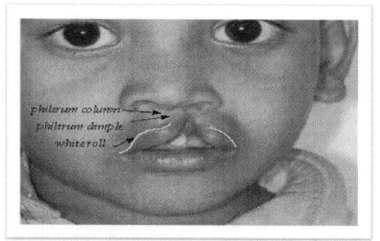

Fig.5ANATOMY OF CLEFT LIPThe Millard procedure for the incomplete unilateral cleft

lip closure

In incomplete clefts most of the time there is less overall distortion of the lip architecture, therefore it is easier to achieve a result close to 'perfection'. Most of the time the rotational incision is extensive, due to the shortness of the NC side. It should have the shape of a fish hook with the tip at landmark (14).

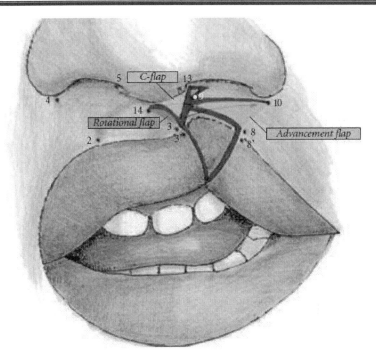

*Fig.6 Landmarks and cutting design
for the Millard procedure.[225]*

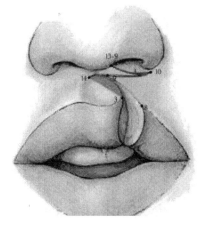

Fig. 7 The Millard procedure just before the closing procedure.[225]

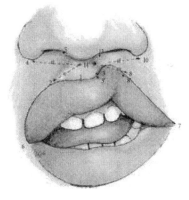

Fig. 8 Landmarks for the Millard design.[225]

Nasal landmarks

Landmark 5 and 13 First mark the end of the medial crus of the lower lateral cartilage. This landmark is considered the columellar base. The German name for this landmark is famous: *'Naseneingangschwelle'*. This is landmark (5) on the non-cleft side and landmark (13) on the cleft side.[225]

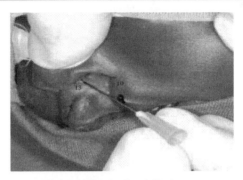

*Fig.9 Marking landmark 13, the
end of the medial crus of
the lower lateral cartilage.*

Landmark 4 and 10 Mark the *alar bases* as landmarks (4) and (10). These landmarks are found at the end of the light reflection on the nostrils. It is most important that both landmarks are in a comparable position right to left, otherwise your measurements are meaningless.

These four landmarks are made close to the cartilage in order to allow for maximum rotation of the alar base. Vermillion border landmarks[225]

Landmark 2, 3 and 1 Landmark (2) is the top of the Cupid's bow on the healthy side and is easy to locate. Therefore it is tattooed right away. Landmark (3) is the end of the white roll on the NCS, it represents the other end of the Cupid's bow. Landmark 3 is tattooed as well. Landmark (1) is chosen as the middle of (2) and (3). It represents the middle of the Cupid's bow.[225]

Landmark 8 On the lateral or cleft side (CS) of the cleft we still need to establish the peak of the Cupid's bow. This landmark (8) is again the end of the white roll on the lateral side. The distance between the commissure on the non-cleft side and the Cupid's bow landmark (6)-(2) is measured and transferred to the cleft side just to check. Often the available distance (7)-(8) is shorter, but in partial clefts this is no rule.[225]

Landmark 3' and 8' On both sides of the cleft landmarks (3) and (8) are the paring peaks of the Cupid's bow and they are marked twice: One landmark is marked just above the white roll (3 and 8) and one landmark is perpendicular to the white roll just in the red lip (3' and 8'). The distance between both upper and lower landmarks is on average 1,5 mm. It is most important that this little distance is equal on both sides. These four cardinal landmarks should stay clearly visible during the whole surgery. Suturing these landmarks at the end of the procedure will create the new Cupid's bow top with a close to normal white roll, in a continuous mode and without steps[225].

Landmarks for the rotational and advancement flap

*Landmark 14*Landmark (14) represents the end of the rotational flap. This landmark is situated about 1 mm caudal to the columella-philtrum-border and in the middle of it.[22]

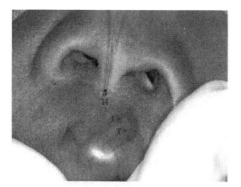

Fig.10Landmark (14) 1 mm caudal of the columella-philtrum border.

Landmark 9 Landmark (9) represents the tip of the advancement flap. To determine the position of landmark (9) you have to measure distance d (14 to 4) and distance (14 to 2). These distances are transposed to the affected sides: distanced starting at landmark 10, distance e starting at landmark (8). Thus landmark (9) is found.[225]

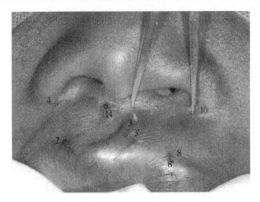

Fig.11 Determining the position
of landmark 9 by transposing
distance 14-4.

Mucosal triangle landmarks

The next effort in design is dedicated to the symmetry and natural fullness of the mucosal part of the lip, with a symmetrical flowing of dry and wet tissues. ***Wet-dry border*** First, determine the wet-dry border. Mark these lines, on both sides, with the wooden stick dipped in methylene blue.[225]

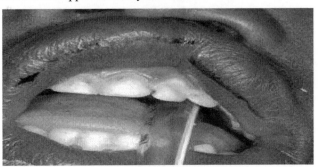

Fig.12Marking of the wet-dry
border.

The distance from landmark (2) to (A) should finally become the lipmucosa length on the side of the cleft too. Distance (3)-(B1) is too small, compared to (2)-(A), therefore a triangular piece of mucosa is taken from the cleft side and is brought in via a deep incision to the opposite side. Since length (3)-(B1) is 'x' shorter than (2)-(A), 'x' must be added to establish equal length[225.]

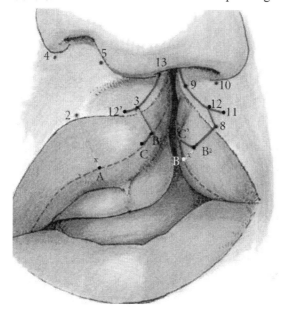

Fig.13 Landmarks for the mucosal
triangle (the illustration isfrom Tennison-Randallprocedure but the principalis the same for the Millard).

Landmark A and B Measure the distance between landmark (2) and the wet-dry border in a perpendicular fashion. This distance (2)-(A) is the reference for the pair side(there is no need to tattoo landmark A). The same distance is measured on the CS lip from (8) to the wet-dry border. This is most often not done in a perpendicular way since the lip is often thinner near this side, so (B) is chosen more laterally on the CS lip. This landmark (B) is clearly indicated with a needle dipped in methylene blue.[225]

Landmark B1 and B2 Then measure the distance from landmark (3) perpendicular to the blue line and tattoo landmark (B1). Deduct this distance (3)-(B1) from distance (8)-(B)to find landmark (B2).

Landmark C and C' Choose landmark (C') on the wet dry border on the cleft side in such a way you create a more-or-less equally sided mucosal triangle. Create landmark (C) on the wet-dry border on the non-cleft side, on such a distance from (B1) that the mucosal triangle will nicely fit in—approximately the distance (B)-(B2). Distance (B)-(B2) is the base of an equal-sided triangle, with one side of the triangle lying along the blue line. This full body mucosa-muscle triangle, after incision, will be brought in a deep incision from (B1) to (C), thus splitting (B1). Later, the upper half of (B1) will be sutured to (B2), the lower half to (B). Landmark (C') will be sutured to (C). When this is done appropriately the lip comes close to symmetry and natural fullness.[225]

Infiltration

Infiltration is started in the lip and nose with local anesthesia/adrenaline. To enlarge dimensions and prevent bleeding of the superior labial artery, pump the lips up quite firmly (2-3cc). For good vasoconstriction wait 5-10 minutes. Use this time to make your 'cutting design' by connecting the marking landmarks.

Cutting design

The cutting design is made with methylene blue and the wooden stick. Connect most of the tattooed landmarks as shown in the illustrations. Pay attention and be conservative in the tissues you disregard, especially on the mucosa-skin borders[225]

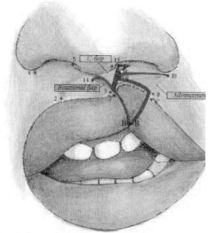

Fig.14 Cutting design and directionsin which flaps shouldbe transposed.
In this fig.the mucosaltriangle is not madebecause the volumes of thered lip fit (distance 3-B1 =8-B).

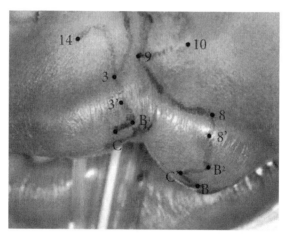

Fig.15 Picture of the cutting design.In this case the mucosaltriangle wasnecessary.

Rotational flap With the wood stick start drawing from landmark (3) towards landmark (14).Close to the columella base the drawing curves medially, clearly flirting with the columella-philtrum border, then it goes downward to the mid-landmark(14). Make sure the curve is wide enough (about 2 mm). It should look like a little fish bracket. A too narrow curve prohibits sufficient rotation of your rotation flap.[225]

C flap Near the columella, between the rotational flap and advancement flap is a no man's land of tissue and skin. Part of it is the C flap, the rest is some extra tissue, most of it mucosa. One limb of the C flap is constituted by the rotational incision, the other one by the line connecting landmark (13) and landmark (3). The upper half of landmark (9) will be sutured to (13). To be able to do this a little dog ear triangle has to be excised. The C flap comes in between this little flap and the advancement flap helping to create the nostril sill. Sometimes you'll have to cut off the tip of the C flap because it's too long—this is part of the cut-as-you-go.[225]

Cutting

Cutting of the mucosal and cutaneous tissues for the cutting procedure, use blade 11. Make no incision deeper than the submucosal or subcutaneous layer. This way there is no undue damage to the orbicular muscles. Remove the mucosal and cutaneous tissues in a conservative way. Always have in mind your blue tattoo landmarks, and leave them in the not-to-be-removed part.

Save as much tissue as possible. Use at least three fresh blades no. 11 for a single surgery, or combine the 11 blade with 15 blades. When cutting the rotation flap make the curve wide enough and fluent. There should be no 'corners'.[225]

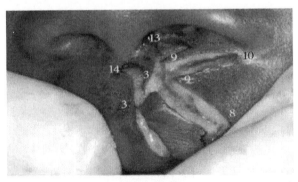

Fig.16 Cutting procedure. The initialincision is no deeperthan the submucosal orsubcutaneous layer.

Cutting for the Basket-Weave Muscle Repair

We believe the muscle inter digitating technique rests on a sound surgical basis and greatly helps to harmonize the lip structures where it is most stigmatizing: the muscular layer. Its promise, indeed, is to create an un disturbed functional and anatomical fair muscular unit around the 'once cleft' mouth. Start with a through and through incision separating the orbicular muscle in a caudal muscle part belonging to the mucosal lip and a cranial muscle part belonging to the skin part of the lip. This is done importantly at the level of the white roll. For the moment we leave the caudal muscle part untouched.[225]

Dissect the cranial muscle part from the skin and the mucosa over a distance of 10 mm on the CS and 5 mm on the NCS. Do this in one cutting movement ,fixing the lip firmly between thumb and index finger. Take special attention to free the muscle completely from the nasal spine on the NCS and from the alar base near the CS. You can use a dental periosteal (molt no. 9) to achieve this to its full extent. Cut the undermined cranial part of the muscle into 3 equal slices.[225]

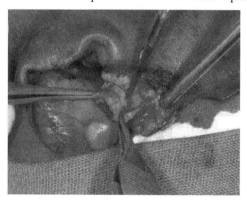

Fig.17 The cranial part of the orbicular
muscle before it iscut (the illustration is from the Tennison-Randall procedure
but the prinicipal isthe same for the Millard).

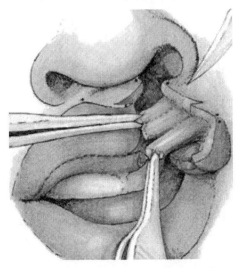

Fig.18 Cutting the orbicular musclein three equal slices (theillustration is from the Tennison-Randall procedurebut the prinicipal is thesame for the Millard).

Undermining of the alar base area

Alar base area The alar base area can easily be reached from underneath the cranial muscle part. Release the alar pad from the alveolus with a pair of scissors and a molt no. Elevate the soft tissues from the pyriform aperture in the supra-periosteal plane. Follow the pyriform aperture on the CS over the periosteum with a pair of scissors and undermine the cheek area until the cleft can be closed with no, or minimal, tension. Be careful not to damage the infraorbital nerve. Protect the nerve by putting your index finger on the infraorbital foramen.[225]

In partial cleft lips this undermining should not be too extensive. Adequate undermining means that the advancement flap can be moved into the rotational gap with no tension. This should be checked with a single hook on landmark (8) and (3) to pull landmark (3) up, thus opening the space that should receive the advancement flap. This should bring both sides together without tension.[225]

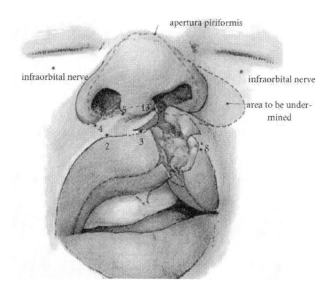

Fig.19 Undermining the alar basearea.(The illustration is from a Tennison procedure but theprinciple is the same for the Millard.)

Lower lateral cartilage At this moment you might free the lower lateral cartilage on the affected side from the overlying skin with a blunt curved pair of scissors. If you do this, at the end of the operation you should excoriate the lower lateral cartilage and fixate it to the skin using mattress sutures. We tend not to do this in small babies because it causes unnecessary damage to the cartilage. We prefer to do a secondary rhinoplasty at a later stage.[225]

Suturing.

Try-in of the suture for the alar base positioning

Position the alar base using a vicryl 5-0. This suture is important for two reasons. It levels both nostrils on the same height and it determines the width of the nostril. Pick up the areolar tissue directly under the alar base (10), with the PDS needle and come out exactly underneath landmark (9). Stay in the tissue, don't come out through the skin. Then pass the needle through the columellar base (13). Come out through the skin at its homologue landmark (5). Return from landmark (5), but in a slightly different direction in order to have some tissue in the loop[225]

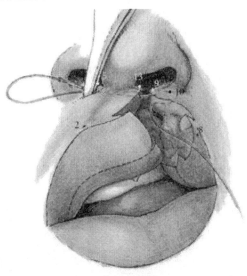

Fig.20 Try-in suture for the alarbase positioning.(The illustration is from aTennison-Randall procedurebut the principle is thesame for the Millard.)

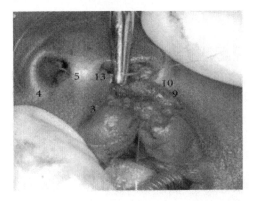

Fig.21.Passing the needle throughthe columellar base.

Now examine the result by temporarily tying the suture. This is the moment to accept or possibly redo the suture by carefully examining the 3-dimensional position of the alar base on the affected side (in the axial plane and the coronal plane).[225]

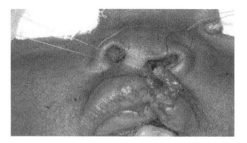

*Fig.22Examining the position of
the alar base after temporarily
tying the suture.*

If the suture seems fine, re-open the knot and attach a mosquito clamp to both ends of the suture. The knot is to be finished at a later stage of the surgery, after the oral vestibule and the floor of the nose are sutured, otherwise access to the oral vestibule and floor of the nose will become difficult.[225]

Vestibular suturing

In partial clefts there is too much mucosa on the inside of the lip so you'll have to excise some of it, creating a V-shape with legs of equal length. Close the defect using a vicryl 5-0 stit.[225]

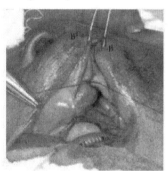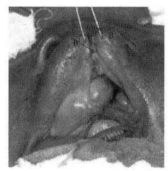

Fig.23 The suturing of the mucosalpart of the lip.

Nasal floor suturing

In partial clefts the floor of the nose is always too wide and a wedge of tissue needs to be excised. Close the wedge by suturing landmark (9) to (13).

Alar base suturing

Now is the moment to make the knot in the previously placed suture of the alar base.

Basket-weave muscle suturing

In order to give the lip a more natural dynamic, as during whistling, we will attach the muscular slings to the sub-dermal layer as it is at the normal side. To suture the cranial muscle layer, draw two vertical lines on the non-affected side to show where the muscle slings are attached to the skin. It can see where the muscles are attached to the skin. Mirror these two vertical lines to

the affected side. The muscle slings from the CS are sutured against the sub-dermal layer on the NCS in three levels and vice versa. To mark these three levels divide the two lines on the affected side in equal parts. The suturing of the muscle slings is carried out using maxon 5-0 (resorbable mono filament). Pick-up the upper muscle sling from the CS, go through the skin of the NCS in one direction, and come back through the same hole but in a different direction, in order to have some subcutaneous tissue inside your loop. Now pick up the upper muscle sling from the NCS and attach it in a similar way to the opposite site. Repeat the same procedure for the middle and lower muscle slings.[225]

Caudal muscle layer suturing

After having sutured all six muscle slings, suture the caudal muscle layer belonging to the red part of the lip. Do this with a vicryl 4-0 stitch going through the cranial part of the muscle parallel to and just below the white roll, with the knot on the deep side. This should bring the Cupid's bow and white roll in an exact pleasing position. Landmark (3) and (8) should come close together, as well as (3') and (8'). If not, reconsider the stitch. There is no need to tighten the knot firmly, since this can disturb the flow of the skin suturing.[225]

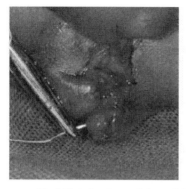
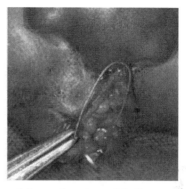

Fig.24Suturing the caudal musclelayer belong to the red partof the lip.
Final closure suturing

Incision mucosal triangle

To receive the *mucosal triangle,* make an incision from (B) to (C). This incision is always along the wet-dry border.

Subcutaneous sutures-Now use vicryl 5-0 subcutaneous sutures to bring the skin flaps into their correct positions. Start with a subcutaneous suture at the *Cupid's bow* landmark (3) and (8).

Also place a subcutaneous suture under the tip of the *C-flap* and the *advancement flap.* Making both of these subcutaneous stitches should give you a sensation of relief and joy, as the wound edges over the whole line fall naturally and fluently.[225]

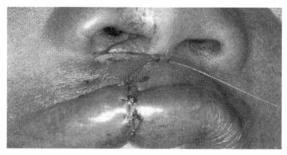

Fig.25 Suturing the tip of the advancement flap.

Back cut If you see that landmark (3) is still being pulled up because the rotation flap is too short you can lengthen it by making a very small back cut starting at marking point (14) coming vertically downward. If you go laterally this will influence the width of the nostrils. Keep in mind that a back cut of 0.5 mm will lengthen the rotation flap by 1 mm.

Skin suturing Suture the skin with catgut 6-0. If you have the opportunity to remove the sutures after 5 or 6 days, you might prefer to use nylon 6-0.

Mucosal triangle Suture the mucosal triangle with vicryl 5-0 into the opening in the wet-dry border. Finish by suturing the rest of the mucosal lip.[225]

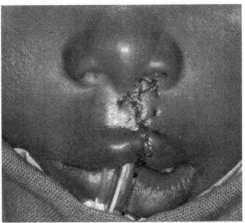

Fig.26 nice result.The invagination point are due to the basket weavetechnique. They fade awayin a week time.

Silastic sheet suturing

You could suture a little roll of silastic sheet into the operated nostril and fix it to the septum with a PDS mattress suture. Leave it in place until the PDS has resorbed and the sheet comes out by itself. The sheet will support the lower lateral cartilage to obtain a more rounded nostril.

MODIFICATIONS OF ROTATION-ADVANCEMENT REPAIR

MILLARD II OPERATION

Adequate rotation has been a problem for a number of surgeons. Millard himself suggested a remedy, including an acute back-cut at approximately 90° at the end of the rotation incision, running parallel but medial to the philtrum, and the C flap insertion into the upper half of the back-cut. During the final suturing, the tip of the advancement flap is sutured to the depth of the rotation back-cut. This increases the rotation and ensures adequate lengthening and horizontalisation of the cupid's bow.

SKOOG'S TECHNIQUE

Skoog (1958) used a small, inferior triangular inter-digitation across the philtrum base in addition to the regular rotation. This procedure has the advantage of allowance for increase in the lip length, but creates a horizontal scar across the philtrum.

MOHLER'S MODIFICATION

Mohler (1986) extended the rotation into the base of the columella, made a back-cut, and sutured it to the lateral flap.

OTHER TECHNIQUES

TENNISON-RANDALL TRIANGULAR FLAP

None of the techniques designed to correct the cleft lip deformity until the 1950s recognised the existence of the cupid's bow on the cleft side of the midline. *Tennison in 1952* demonstrated a triangular flap repair that preserved the cupid's bow for the first time. He inserted a wedge from the lateral lip into the lower portion of the medial lip, and achieved good results. *Tennison* called this technique 'the stencil method'. *Randall in 1971* modified the technique by making the triangular flap smaller, and defined the mathematics of the method.[225]

While this technique allows muscle dissection to achieve functional approximation and preserves the cupid's bow, the philtrum is broken by the triangular flap and secondary correction is difficult. Also, mathematical precision in measurement is necessary in the pre-operative assessment and during the surgery. Even though more sophisticated technique have since been described, the *Tennison-Randall method* remains popular with a number of surgeons, especially in the correction of incomplete clefts.[22]

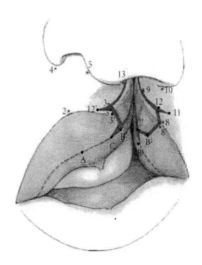

Fig.27 Cutting design for the Tennison-Randall procedure

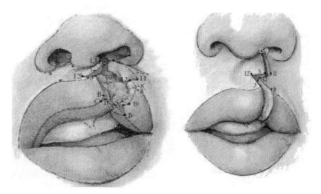

Fig.28 Tennison-Randall procedure after cutting

Land marks

Nasal and vermillion border landmarks for the Tennison-Randall design

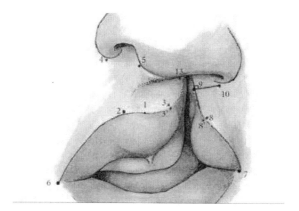

Fig 29.Tennison-Randall just before
closure of the skin and mucosa.

Nasal landmarks

Landmark 5 and 13 First mark the end of the medial crus of the lower lateral cartilage. This landmark is considered the columellar base. The German name for this landmark is famous: *'Naseneingangschwelle'*. This is landmark (5) on the non-cleft side and landmark (13) on the cleft side.[225]

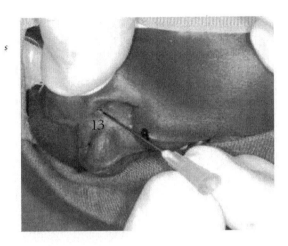

Fig 30.Marking landmark 13 at the end of the medial crus of the lower lateral cartilage.

Landmark 4 and 10 Mark the alar bases as landmarks (4) and (10). These landmarks are found at the end of the light reflection on the nostrils. It is most important that both landmarks are in a comparable position right to left, otherwise your measurements are meaningless.

These four landmarks are made close to the cartilage in order to allow for maximum rotation of the alar base.[225]

Vermillion border landmarks

Landmark 2, 3 and 1 Landmark (2) is the top of the Cupid's bow on the healthy side and is easy to locate. Therefore it is tattooed right away. Landmark (3) is the end of the white roll on the NCS, it represents the other end of the Cupid's bow. Landmark 3 is tattooed as well. Landmark (1) is chosen as the middle of (2) and (3). It represents the middle of the Cupid's bow.[225]

Landmark 8 On the lateral or cleft side (CS) we still need to establish the peak of the Cupid's bow. This is landmark (8) and is the end of the white roll on the CS. The distance between the commissure on the non-cleft side and the Cupid's bow landmark (6)-(2) is measured and transferred to the cleft side. Almost universally the available distance (7)-(8) is shorter. This gives an idea of the amount of shortening of the lip on the CS.[225]

Landmark 3' and 8'On both sides of the cleft landmarks (3) and (8) are the paring peaks of the Cupid's bow and they are marked twice: One landmark is marked just above the white roll (3 and 8) and one landmark is perpendicular to the white roll just in the red lip (3' and 8'). The distance between both upper and lower landmarks is on average 1,5 mm. It is most important that this little distance is equal on both sides. These four cardinal landmarks should stay clearly visible during the whole surgery. Suturing these landmarks at the end of the procedure will create the new Cupid's bow top with a close to normal white roll, in a continuous mode and without steps.[225]

Skin triangle landmarks

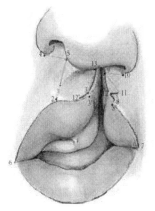

Fig31 Measurements for the triangular design

The distance from landmark (5) to (2) should finally become the lip length on the cleft-side too. Since length (13)-(3) is 'x' shorter than (5)-(2), 'x' must be added to establish equal length. We bring this in as a triangular skin flap from the cleft side with a base of 'x'.[225]

This triangular skin flap, after incision, will be brought in via a deep incision from (3) to (12'), thus splitting (3). Later, the upper half of (3) will be sutured to (11), the lower half to (8). This reconstructs the lip with a normal contoured Cupid's bow and a zigzag scar line, which also prevents vertical scar contracture.[225]

Landmark 11 Landmark (11) is situated at a distance 'x' from landmark (8) perpendicularly away from the white roll.

Landmark 9 Landmark (9) is paramount because it defines two structures on the affected side: the width of the nostril and the length of the lip. Landmark (9) should be located on a distance (3)-(13) from landmark (11),on the border between skin and mucosa. This distance determines in part the length of the lip.

Also the distance from the alar base (10) to landmark (9) should be identical to the distance (4)-(5) on the normal side. This will determine the width of the new nostril. Indeed landmark (9) will be sutured to landmark (13).For the nostril landmark (9) is ideally situated on a perpendicular line from the alar base on the affected side to the border between skin and mucosa and exactly on this border.

Landmark 12 and 12' Finally we mark a third landmark (12). It is facing the cleft and is the top of the more-or-less 'equally sided triangle'. This landmark should be chosen as close to the vermillion border as possible, in order to save as much skin as possible. The homologue landmark on the NCS is (12'), located just above the white roll on a distance x from (3).[225]

Mucosal triangle landmarks

The next effort in design is dedicated to the symmetry and natural fullness of the mucosal part of the lip, with a symmetrical flowing of dry and wet tissues. **Wet-dry border** First, determine the wet-dry border. Mark these lines, on both sides, with the wooden stick dipped in methylene blue[225]

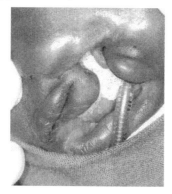

Fig 32 Marking of the wet-dry border.

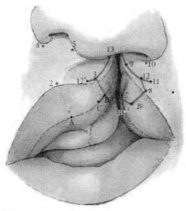

Fig 33.Measurements done to obtain symmetrical volumes of the mucosal part of the lip.

The distance from landmark (2) to (A) should finally become the lip mucosa length on the side of the cleft too. Distance (3)-(B1) is too small, compared to (2)-

(A), therefore a triangular piece of mucosa is taken from the cleft side and is brought in via a deep incision to the opposite side. Since length (3)-(B1) is'x' shorter than (2)-(A), 'x' must be added to establish equal length.[225]

Landmark A and B measured the distance between landmark (2) and the wet-dry border in a perpendicular fashion. This distance (2)-(A) is the reference for the pair side (there is no need to tattoo landmark A). The same distance is measured on the CS lip from (8) to the wet-dry border. This is most often not done in a perpendicular way since the lip is often thinner near this side, so (B) is chosen more laterally on the CS lip. This landmark (B) is clearly indicated with a needle dipped in methylene blue.[225]

Landmark B1 and B2 Then measure the distance from landmark (3) perpendicular to the blue line and tattoo landmark (B1). Deduct this distance (3)-(B1) from distance (8)-(B) to find landmark (B2).[225]

Landmark C and C' Choose landmark C' on the wet dry border on the cleft side in such a way you create a more-or-less equally sided mucosal triangle. Create landmark C on the wet-dry border on the non-cleft side, on such a distance from (B1) that the mucosal triangle will nicely fit in—approximately the distance (B)-(B2). Distance (B)-(B2) is the base of an equal-sided triangle, with one side of the triangle lying along the blue line. This full body mucosa-muscle triangle, after incision, will be brought in a deep incision from (B1) to (C), thus splitting (B1). Later, the upper half of (B1) will be sutured to (B2), the lower half to (B). Landmark (C') will be sutured to (C). When this is done appropriately the lip comes close to symmetry and natural fullness.[225]

Vestibular landmarks

Landmark TV and TV' To complete our design we need to tattoo two more landmarks: the vestibular tops on both sides of the cleft—where the alveolar process starts. On the NCS, this is landmark (TV). On the cleft side we mark the same landmark as(TV'). This landmark, though, is more arbitrary than landmark (TV).[225]

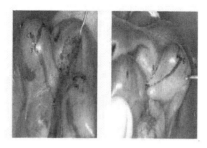

Fig34. Landmark TV (non-cleft side) and TV' (cleft side).

Infiltration Infiltration is started in the lip and nose with local anesthesia/adrenaline. To enlarge dimensions and prevent bleeding of the superior labial artery, pump the lips up quite firmly (2-3cc). For good vasoconstriction wait 5-10 minutes. Use this time to make your 'cutting design' by connecting the landmarks.[225]

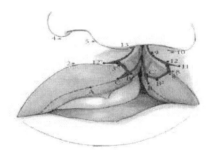

Fig 35.Cutting design for the Tennison-Randall procedure.

The cutting design is made with methylene blue and the wooden stick.

Muco-philtral design Connect most of the tattooed landmarks as shown in the illustration. Pay attention and be conservative in the tissues you disregard, especially on the mucosa-skin borders.[225]

Muco-nasal design NCS From landmark (13), the Naseneingangschwelle, continue the design to the top of the oral vestibule (TV). For this, follow the border between the nasal skin and the oral mucosa, distinctive in color and texture. From (TV) the drawing is completed, returning along the wet-dry border to finally reach (B1).[225]

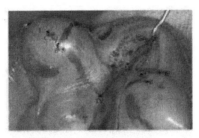

Fig.36 Cutting design for the anterior part of the nose on the non-cleft side.

Muco-nasal design CS From landmark (9) continue the design deeper in the nose along the border of the nasal skin and the oral mucosa. The end is (TV'), the top of the alveolar process on the cleft side. In order to be able to join the pair sides (TV) to (TV'), a small back cut inside the nose is necessary. Also some undermining is necessary along the line (9) to (TV') in order to bring (TV') to (TV) bridging the cleft gap. At the NCS undermining is almost impossible, therefore we do the undermining on the CS. This incision is also continued along the wet-dry border to reach landmark (B).[225]

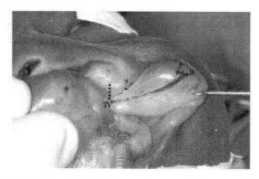

Fig 37Cutting design for the anterior part of the nose on the cleft side.

Cutting

Cutting of the mucosal and cutaneous tissues

For the cutting procedure, use blade 11. Make no incision deeper than the Sub-mucosal or subcutaneous layer. This way there is no undue damage to the orbicular muscles. Remove the mucosal and cutaneous tissues in a conservative way. Always have in mind your blue tattoo landmarks, and leave them in the not-to-be-removed part.   Save as much tissue as possible. Use at least three fresh blades no. 11 for asingle surgery, or combine the 11 blade with 15 blades.

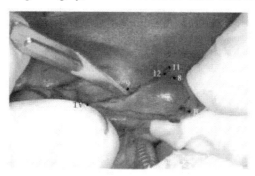

Fig38.Initial incision no deeper than submucosal or subcutaneous layer

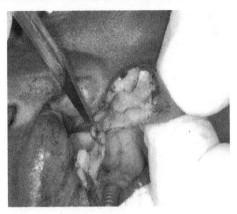

Fig 39.Removal of the mucosal
tissues.

Cutting for the Basket-Weave Muscle Repair

We believe the muscle interdigitating technique rests on a sound surgical basis and greatly helps to harmonize the lip structures where it is most stigmatizing: the muscular layer. Its promise, indeed, is to create an undisturbed functional and anatomical fair muscular unit around the 'once cleft' mouth. Start with a through and through incision separating the orbicular muscle in a caudal muscle part belonging to the mucosal lip and a cranial muscle part belonging to the skin part of the lip. This is done importantly at the level of the white roll. For the moment we leave the caudal muscle part untouched.[225]

Dissect the cranial muscle part from the skin and the mucosa over a distance of 10 mm on the CS and 5 mm on the NCS. Do this in one cutting movement, fixing the lip firmly between thumb and index finger. Take special attention to free the muscle completely from the nasal spine on the NCS and from the alar base near the CS. You can use a dental periosteal (molt no. 9) to achieve this to its full extent. Cut the undermined cranial part of the muscle into 3 equal slices.[225]

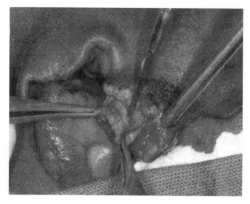

Fig 40The cranial part of the orbicular muscle after dissection and before it is cut

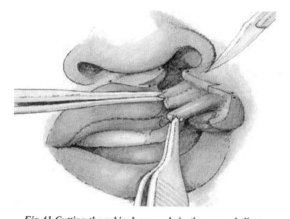

Fig 41.Cutting the orbicular muscle in three equal slices.

Undermining of the alar base area

Alar base area The alar base area can easily be reached from underneath the cranial muscle part. Release the alar pad from the alveolus with a pair of scissors and a molt no. 9. Elevate the soft tissues from the pyriform aperture in the supraperiosteal plane. Follow the pyriform aperture on the CS over the periosteum with a pair of scissors and undermine the cheek area until the cleft can be closed with

126

no, or minimal, tension. Be careful not to damage the infraorbital nerve. Protect the nerve by putting your index finger on the infraorbital foramen.[225]

Lower lateral cartilage At this moment you might free the lower lateral cartilage on the affected side from the overlying skin with a blunt curved pair of scissors. If you do this, at the end of the operation you should exorotate the lower lateral cartilage and fixate it to the skin using mattress sutures. We tend not to do this in small babies because it causes unnecessary damage to the cartilage. We prefer to do a secondary rhinoplasty at a later stage.[225]

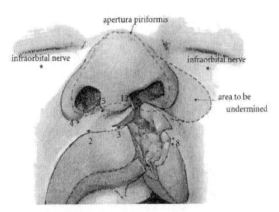

Fig 42.Undermining of the alar base area.

Suturing

Try-in of the suture for the alar base positioning .Position the alar base using a PDS 5-0. This suture is important for two reasons. It levels both nostrils on the same height and it determines the width of the nostril. Pick up the areolar tissue directly under the alar base (10), with the PDS needle and come out exactly underneath landmark (9). Stay in the tissue, don't come out through the skin. Then pass the needle through the columellar base (13). Come out through the skin at its homologue landmark(5). Return from landmark (5), but in a slightly different direction in order to have some tissue in the loop.[225]

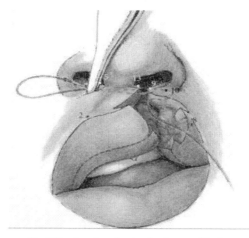

Fig.43 Try-in suture for the alar base positioning.

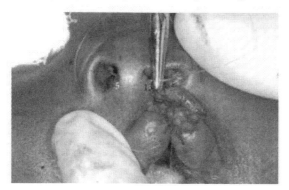

Fig44 Passing the needle through the columellar base.

Now examine the result by temporarily tying the suture. This is the moment to accept or possibly redo the suture by carefully examining the 3-dimensional position of the alar base on the affected side (in the axial plane and the coronal plane)[225].

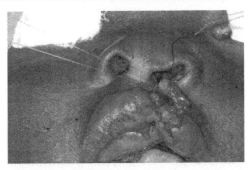

Fig 45.Examining the position of the alar base after temporarily

tying the suture.

If the suture seems fine, re-open the knot and attach a mosquito clamp to both ends of the suture.[225] The knot is to be finished at a later stage of the surgery, after the oral vestibule and the floor of the nose are sutured, otherwise access to the oral vestibule and floor of the nose will become difficult[225].

Vestibular suturing

Vestibular border Start first to make an incision from (TV') along the vestibular border, as long as needed to cross the cleft-gap without tension. Dissect this part of the vestibularmucosa. This incision in the vestibule releases the alar pad area from the alveolus.

Landmark (TV') of the CS finally has to be sutured to landmark (TV) on the NCS. To make this possible without tension start more laterally along the vestibular mucosa incision to put 2 or 3 intermediate sutures using vicryl 5-0or polysorb 5-0.[225]

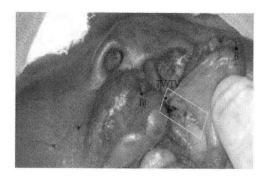

Fig 46.Suturing of TV to TV'.

Vestibular lip Then continue the suturing of the mucosal part of the lip from TV/TV' up to the wet-dry border (landmark B1 and B).[225]

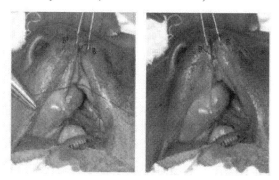

Fig 47 .The suturing of the mucosal part of the lip.

Nasal floor suturing

The suturing of the anterior floor of the nose always starts posterior and proceeds anterior.

The nasal mucosa from landmark (9) to (TV') on the CS needs to be undermined and released and often there is a need for a right angled back-cut starting from (TV') lateral towards the lower concha in order to gain sufficient nasal mucosal tissue. Start from the previously sutured TV/TV' and proceed anterior, with two or three stitches, to finally suture landmark (13) to (9).[225]

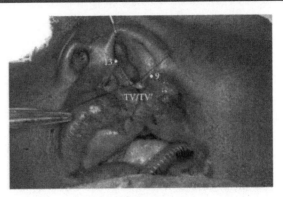

Fig 48.Nasal floor suturing.

Alar base suturing

Now is the moment to make the knot in the previously placed suture of the alar base.

Basket-weave muscle suturing

In order to give the lip a more natural dynamic, as during whistling, we will attach the muscular slings to the sub dermal layer as it is at the normal side.

To suture the cranial muscle layer, draw two vertical lines on the non-affected side to show where the muscle slings are attached to the skin. You can see where the muscles are attached to the skin. Mirror these two vertical lines to the affected side. The muscle slings from the CS are sutured against the sub-dermal layer on the NCS in three levels and vice versa. To mark these three levels divide the two lines on the affected side in equal parts.[225]

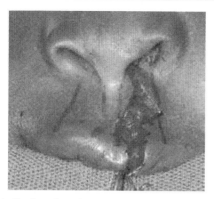

Fig.49 Vertical lines indicating where the muscle slings should be attached to the skin.

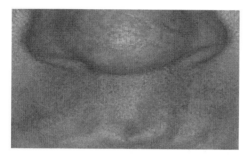

Fig .50 Normal lip during whistling. You can see where the muscle is attached to the skin.

The suturing of the muscle slings is carried out using maxon 5-0 (resorbable mono filament). Pick-up the upper muscle sling from the CS, go through the skin of the NCS in one direction, and come back through the same hole but in a different direction, in order to have some subcutaneous tissue inside your loop. Now pick up the upper muscle sling from the NCS and attach it in a similar way to the opposite site.[225]

Skin incision triangle Before suturing the lower muscle sling make the deep skin incision from landmark (3) to (12') in order to receive the triangular flap. If not, you risk cutting the lower muscle sling suture. The direction of this incision is parallel just above the white roll. Others prefer to direct the incision more into the skin and away from the white roll.[225]

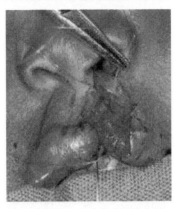

Fig.51 Going through the skin in one direction, and coming back through the same holein a different direction

Repeat the same procedure for the middle and lower muscle slings

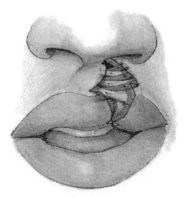

Fig 52 -The basket-weave muscle repair.

Caudal muscle layer suturing

After having sutured all six muscle slings, suture the caudal muscle layer belonging to the red part of the lip. Do this with a vicryl 5-0 stitch going through the cranial part of the muscle Parallel to and just below the white roll, with the knot on the deep side. This should bring the Cupid's bow and white roll in an exact pleasing position. Landmarks (3) and (8) should come close together, as well as (3') and (8'). If

133

not, reconsider the stitch. There is no need to tighten the knot firmly, since this can disturb the flow of the skin suturing.

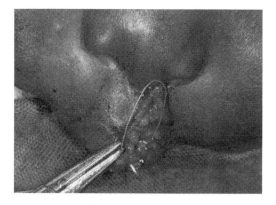

Fig 53 *Suturing the caudal muscle layer belong to the red part of the lip.*

Final closure suturing

Incisions for triangles As indicated the incision on the NCS to receive the skin triangle should bed one before the suturing of the lower basket sling. To receive the mucosal triangle, make an incision from (B) to (C'). This incision is always along the wet-dry border.[225]

Subcutaneous sutures Now use vicryl 5-0 subcutaneous sutures to bring the skin flaps into their correct positions. Start with a subcutaneous suture at the Cupid's bow landmark (3) and (8). Another important subcutaneous suture is one from landmark(11) to (3). Making both of these subcutaneous stitches should give you a sensation of relief and joy, as the wound edges over the whole line finally fall naturally and fluently.[225]

Skin suturing Suture the skin with catgut 6-0 (in developing countries this is still easy toget). If you have the opportunity to remove the sutures after 5 or 6 days, youmight prefer to use nylon 6-0.[225]

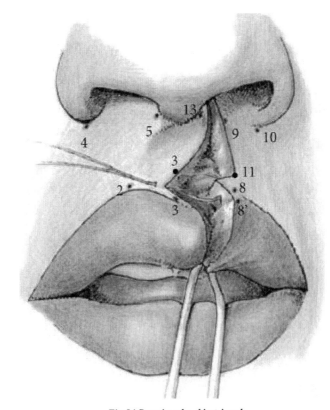

Fig.54 Suturing the skin triangle.

Mucosal triangle Suture the mucosal triangle with vicryl 5-0 into the opening in the wet-dry border. Finish by suturing the rest of the mucosal lip.

Silastic sheet suturing

You could suture a little roll of silastic sheet into the operated nostril and fix it to the septum with a PDS mattress suture. Leave it in place until the PDS has resorbed and the sheet comes out by itself. The sheet will support the lower lateral cartilage to obtain a more rounded nostril.[225]

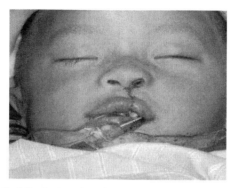

Fig.55 Roll of silastic sheet fixated to the septum inside the operated nostril

DELAIRE'S FUNCTIONAL LIP CLOSURE

Delaire, a French surgeon, in a series of papers from 1971 to 1986 demonstrated what he called a 'functional closure' of cleft lip. This technique does not make use of flaps, and relies essentially on accurate reconstruction of the muscles of the lip and nose. This operation creates a highly symmetric nose and a functional lip. Its main disadvantage is a straight-line scar and inability to achieve adequate lengthening of the lip, resulting in a notching. But its proponents claim that this lack of lip symmetry will gradually reduce by the effect of normal labial muscle function.

BILATERAL CLEFT LIP REPAIR

A lip that is completely cleft on both sides is usually associated with a complete cleft of the palate, but it may involve only the primary palate. The prolabium demonstrates total absence of orbicularis oris muscle, and is attached to the tip of the nose by an almost non-existent columella.

Treatment plane

The pre-treatment evaluation should determine

    (i) Whether the cleft is complete or incomplete

    (ii) The size and position of the premaxilla and the prolabium

    (iii) The length of the columella

    (iv) Whether the inter-alveolar space is sufficient to accommodate the premaxilla

    (v) The presence or absence of associated anomalies, like lip pits.

In any plan of treatment, the following principles should be applied *(Cronin, 1957)*

    a) The prolabium should be used to form the full vertical length of the lip

    b) The thin prolabial lining should be turned down for lining

    c) The central vermilion is built up with the vermilion-muscle flaps from the lateral lip segments

    d) The vermilion ridge should come from the lateral lip segments

e)   No lateral lip skin should be used beneath the prolabium

f)   Reposition of severely protruding premaxilla not only permits earlier and better repair of the lip by relieving undue tension, but also makes one-stage repair possible.

g)   Collapse of the maxillary processes behind the protruding premaxilla requires prevention or expansion with maxillary orthopaedics.

h)   Bone grafting is indicated to stabilise the premaxilla when it is not united on either side. (controversial)

TIMING OF REPAIR

Repair of bilateral cleft lip is generally deferred until the child weighs approximately 12-14 pounds in order to have more tissue to work with. If the premaxilla protrudes excessively and non-surgical methods used for its correction, it is important to begin immediately, so that advantage may be taken of the soft pliable condition of the bones and the rapid growth that takes place during the first few months.

CONTROL OF THE PROTRUDING PREMAXILLA

When the position of the premaxilla is fairly normal or the protrusion is only moderate, the lip can be repaired over it with little tension. But excessive protrusion is a serious complicating factor. Attempts to repair the lip over a conspicuously protruding premaxilla may, because of excessive tension, result either in actual dehiscence of the wound or in spreading of the scar.

The methods currently used in dealing with the prominent premaxilla are

1.   Traction by external elastic with headcap

2.   Closure of the cleft, one side at a time

3. Lip adhesion

4. Intra-oral elastic devices

5. Surgical setback of the premaxilla

The surgical method is seldom indicated. It is used only after all the other methods including lip adhesion has failed. Surgical setback might also be considered in an older child for whom lip repair has not corrected a severely protruding premaxilla.

TECHNIQUES OF BILATERAL CLEFT LIP REPAIR

STRAIGHT LINE CLOSURE (VEAU III OPERATION)

Point 'a' is located medial to the tip of the base of the ala. Point 'c' is placed in the midline of the valley of the Cupid 's bow on the vermilion ridge. The point 'b' is placed 3-mm lateral to the point 'c' on the vermilion ridge. Ideally, the line 'ab' should be of equal length as 'a`b'' marked on the lateral lip segment, but slight shortening may be corrected while suturing. After the marking is completed, 1% lignocaine with 1:2,00,000 epinephrine is injected sparingly into the buccal sulcus, the base of the ala and the columella, the prolabium and the lip.

The lip is fixed firmly against a wooden tongue depressor as a`b` is incised completely through the lip with a no.15 Bard-Parker blade. The incision is made vertical to the skin surface so that there is adequate muscle bulk medial to the incision. The skin between a`b` and the vermilion border is excised. This leaves a raw muscle flap (X flap) on the medial aspect of the lateral lip segment. The same procedure is repeated on the other side to create bilateral symmetrical X flaps. Then, under finger pressure, line ab is incised. If sufficient tissue is available, forked flaps are created lateral to line ab to be banked in the nasal floor, otherwise the skin is excised. The remaining vermilion border and mucosal flaps are turned back to be sutured to the mucosa of the respective lateral lip segment as needed.

The vermilion border is incised on the prolabium from point b to the point b on the other side. The tissue inferior to the b-b line is turned down as flap, leaving a space into which the X flaps are brought to each other. This manoeuvre helps to deepen the labial sulcus. The point a` comes to point a, and b` to b on both sides, and the X flaps are sutured together to create the midline of the flap.

If forked flaps are taken, they are turned 90° into the nasal floor and are banked. A 4-0 plain catgut or 4-0 armed vicryl is used for muscle suturing. The skin sutures are given with 6-0 silk or prolene.

Columellar lengthening

A shortened columella is almost always associated with a complete bilateral cleft lip. Columellar lengthening is usually not attempted at the time of initial lip repair. It has been found that early repair results in downward slippage of the columella and lip over the premaxilla. Lengthening of columella may be done any time after the patient is 2-3 years of age.

Cronin (1958) described a method of advancing skin from the floor of the nose and base of the ala into the columella. *Converse (1957)* also used skin from the floor of the nose. *Millard (1958, 1971)* and associates used a forked flap from the prolabium. *Brauer and Fara (1966)* employed the V-Y principle in the region of wide tip.

MILLARD REPAIR OF COMPLETE BILATERAL CLEFT LIP

Millard (1971) developed a method in which the forked flaps are raised initially and stored for future use while the lip is closed in one stage. A prime requisite of this technique is a fairly large prolabium (if the prolabium is too narrow, a straight-line repair or the Wynn method is more preferable). The lateral vermilion mucosal flaps with the white roll are brought to the midline while the prolabial vermilion is turned downward. Millard also advocated a complete mucosa-muscle to muscle-mucosa behind a philtral strip of prolabium.

As a second stage, a V-Y advancement of the banked flaps on the floor of the nose is employed to lengthen the columella.

MILLARD PROCEDURE FOR COMPLETE REPAIR OF BILETERAL CLEFT LIP

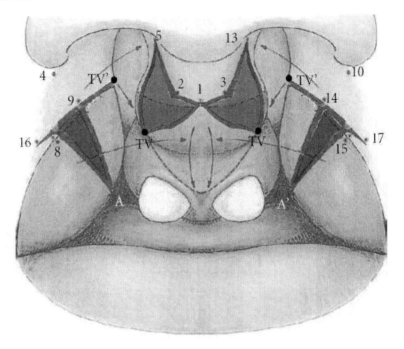

Fig.56Landmarks and cutting design for the bilateral Millardprocedure.

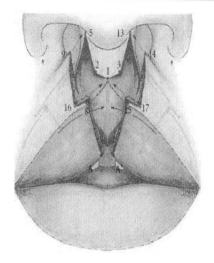

Fig57.Millard procedure after Cutting

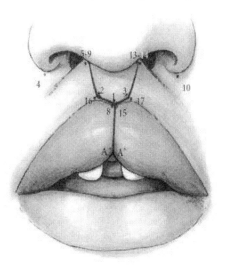

Fig 58 Millard procedure just before closure of the skin andmucosa.

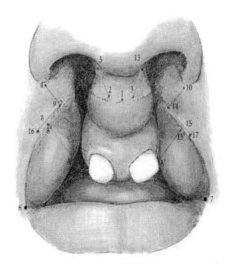

*Fig 59.Landmarks for the bilateral
cleft lip closure according toMillard.*

Nasal landmarks

Landmark 5 and 13: Mark first the end of the medial crus of the lower lateral cartilages on both sides. These landmarks, (5) and (13), are considered as the base of the columella.

The German name for these landmarks is famous: *'Naseneingangschwelle'.*

Landmark 4 and 10: Mark the alar bases (4) and (10). They are found at the end of the light reflectionon the nostrils. Those four landmarks are made close to the cartilage in order to allow for maximum rotation of the alar bases. Otherwise the lower lateral cartilages will remain flattened and the nostrils widened.[225]

Vermillion border landmarks

Landmark 1, 2, 3 mark philtrum middle (1) just at the border between white and red part of the lip. As the philtrum should be no wider than 4 mm you choose philtrum right and left (2) and (3) two mm on both sides next to (1). These last landmarks should be just above the border between the white and red part of the lip. The white roll will be brought in from aside under the philtrum.[225]

143

Landmark 8, 8' and 15, 15'Landmarks (8) and (15) are the end of the white roll at the lateral sides of the clefts. They are marked twice: one landmark is marked just above the white roll and one landmark is perpendicular under the white roll in the red lip. This enables you to cut the white roll in a perpendicular fashion. The distance between both upper and lower landmark is on average 1,5 mm. Most important is that this little distance is equal on both sides. These four cardinal landmarks should stay clearly visible during the whole surgery. Suturing those landmarks at the end of the procedure will create the new white roll under the philtrum, in a continuous mode and without steps. Moreover these landmarks should end up at the same vertical height.[225]

Landmark 16 and 172 mm laterally from landmarks (8) and (15) a landmark is chosen (16) and(17) that at the end of the surgery will be sutured towards (2) and (3).[225]

Landmark 9 and 14 Now the length of the philtrum (5) – (2) is measured and transferred to the lateral side of the cleft starting from landmark (16). There landmark (9) is located just inside the skin along the border between white and red part of the lip. This landmark (9) is to be sutured later on towards (5). Repeat the same procedure on the other side to find landmark (14)[225]

Mucosal triangle landmarks

The next effort in design is dedicated to the symmetry and natural fullness of the mucosal part of the lip, with a symmetrical flowing of dry and wet tissues.

Wet-dry border First, determine the wet-dry border. Mark these lines, on both sides, with the wooden stick dipped in methylene blue.

Landmark A and A' Looking down from landmarks (8) and (15) choose the landmarks (A) and(A') on the wet-dry border in such fashion that the volume of the red part of the lip doesn't diminish towards the middle, thus avoiding a whistling deformity.[225]

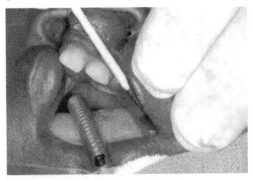

Fig.60 Determining and markingof the wet-dry border.

Landmark A and A'Looking down from landmarks (8) and (15) choose the landmarks (A) and (A') on the wet-dry border in such fashion that the volume of the red part of the lip doesn't diminish towards the middle, thus avoiding a whistling deformity.[225]

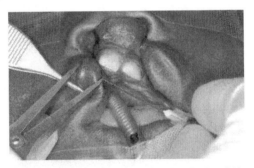

Fig 61.Measuring and tattooing of landmarks A and A'.

Vestibular landmarks

Landmark TV and TV' These landmarks represent the top of the oral vestibule on both sides of the cleft.

Infiltration

Infiltration is started in the lip and nose with local anesthesia/adrenaline. To enlarge dimensions and prevent bleeding of the superior labial artery, pump the lips up quite firmly (2-3cc). For good vasoconstriction wait 5-10 minutes. Use this time to make your 'cutting design' by connecting the marking landmarks.[225]

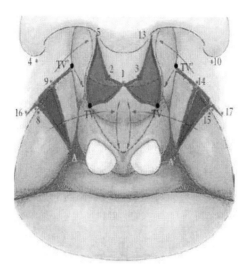

Fig.62 The cutting line design and directions in which flaps will be transposed.

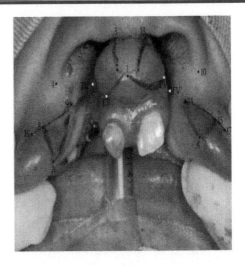

Fig.63 Picture of the cutting design.

Muco-philtral design

Connect all the tattooed landmarks we discussed above. Pay attention to be conservative in the tissues you disregard, especially on the mucosa-skin borders.

Muco-nasal design

Now we still need to draw the mucosal design inside the mucosal cleft lip and nose. Start the design in the anterior part of the nose on the medial sides.Draw a line from landmark (5) to the top of the oral vestibule TV. For this, follow the border of the nasal skin and the nasal mucosa, distinctive in color and texture, towards the oral vestibule.[225]

The oral side of the incision is continued towards landmark (1). On the lateral side, from landmark (9) continue the incision deeper in the nose along the border of the nasal skin and the nasal-oral mucosa to (TV'). Repeat the drawing on the other side of the cleft.[225]

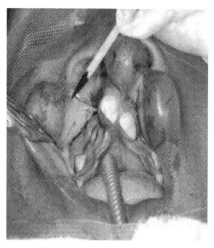

Fig 64 Muco-nasal design.Continuing of the incision from(9) to (TV').

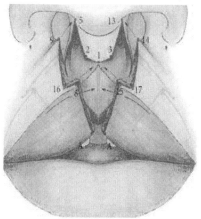

Fig 65 Cutting of the mucosal and cutaneous tissues

For the cutting procedure, use blade 11. Make no incision deeper than the submucosal or subcutaneous layer. This way there is no undue damage to the orbicular muscles. Remove the mucosal and cutaneous tissues in a conservative way. *Always have in mind your blue tattoo landmarks, and leave them in the not-to-be-removed part.* Save as much tissue as possible. Use at least three fresh blades no. 11 for a single surgery, or combine the 11 blade with 15 blades.[225]

Cutting for the Basket-Weave Muscle Repair

We believe the muscle interdigitating technique rests on a sound surgical basis and greatly helps to harmonize the lip structures where it is most stigmatizing: the muscular layer. Its promise, indeed, is to create an undisturbed functional and anatomical fair muscular unit around the 'once cleft' mouth.

Start with a through and through incision separating the orbicular muscle in a caudal muscle part belonging to the mucosal lip and a cranial muscle part belonging to the skin part of the lip. This is done importantly at the level of the white roll. For the moment we leave the caudal muscle part untouched.[225]

Dissect the cranial muscle part from the skin and the mucosa over a distance of 10 mm (10 mm laterally, medially there is no muscle). In the cleft philtrum there is no muscular layer present. So the muscle has to come from the lateral sides. Do this in one cutting movement, fixing the lip firmly between thumb and index finger.[225]

Cut the undermined cranial part of the muscle into 3 equal slices.

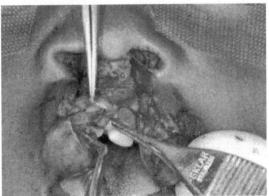

Fig .66Cutting the cranial part of the muscle in 3 equal slices

Undermining of the alar base area

Now undermine the alar base area of the nose on both sides. Follow the pyriform aperture over the periosteum with a pair of scissors and undermine the cheek area till the cleft can be closed with no or minimal tension. Be careful not to damage the infraorbital nerve.[225]

149

Suturing

Try-in of the suture for the alar base positioning

Position the alar base using a PDS 4-0 or 5-0. This suture is important for two reasons. It levels both nostrils on the same height and it determines the width of the nostril.[225] Pick up the areolar tissue directly under the alar base (landmark 10) with the PDS needle and come out exactly at landmark (14). Then pass the needle through landmark (13). Come out at marking point (5) on the other side and pick up the areolar tissue under the second alar base (4) and come out at (9).Return through the philtrum entering at (5) and coming out at (13).

Now examine the result by temporarily tying the suture. This is the moment to accept or possibly redo the suture by carefully examining the 3-dimensional position of the alar bases. If the suture seems fine, re-open the knot and attach a mosquito clamp to both ends of the suture. The knot is to be finished at a later stage of the surgery, after the oral vestibule and the floor of the nose are sutured, otherwise access to the oral vestibule and floor of the nose will become difficult.[225]

Vestibular suturing

Start first to dissect the vestibule of the mouth. The mucosa in the vestibule on the lateral side of the cleft most often needs to be incised and mobilized in order to suture in continuity to the mucosa of the cleft side and across the cleft gap. This is done to the top of the vestibule on the non-cleft side. Start with 2 or 3 intermediate sutures using vicryl 5-0 or polysorb 5-0, each time half way in order to divide the tension.[225]

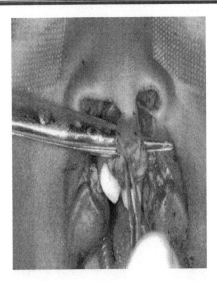

Fig.67 Vestibular incision in order to be able to suture TV to TV'.

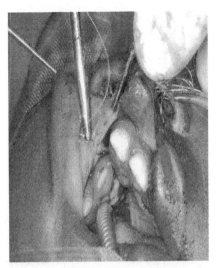

Fig. 68 Intermediate suture to divide the tension to finallysuture TV to TV'.

Then continue the suturing of the mucosal part of the lip along the cleft, up to the wet- dry border (landmark A and A').[225]

Nasal floor suturing

The suturing of the anterior floor of the nose starts from posterior to anterior. Suture landmark (TV') on the lateral side of the cleft to (TV) on the medial side and divide the rest of the distance up to landmark (9) to landmark (5) in 2 or 3 stitches. Do the same on the other side.[225]

Alar base suturing

Now is the moment to make the knot in the previously placed suture of the alar base.

Basket-weave muscle suturing

Now the muscle slings have to be sutured to the skin in such a way that you create a more natural appearance of the lip during whistling. Vertical lines (laterally) and dots (inside the philtrum) are being placed to show where the muscle slings should be attached to the skin.[225]

 Suturing the muscle slings are carried out using maxon 5-0 (resorbable monofilament).Pick up the muscle sling, go through the skin in one direction, and come back through the same hole but in a different direction, in order to havesome subcutaneous tissue inside your loop.[225]

The middle muscle sling on the right side passes through the philtrum andis being sutured to the skin on the lateral side of the cleft on the left side andvice versa. The upper and lower slings on the right side are being sutured to the lateral skin of the philtrum. Same on the left side. show where the muscle slings should be attached to the skin.[225]

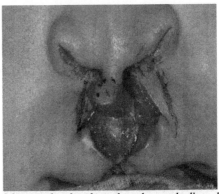

Fig. 69 Vertical lines and dots are placed to show where the muscle slings should be attached to skin

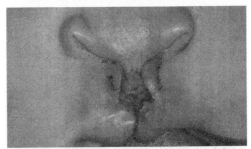

Fig.70   Suturing pattern for the bilateral cleft

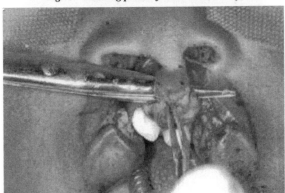

Fig. 71   Hole made to pass the middle muscle slings throughthe philtrum

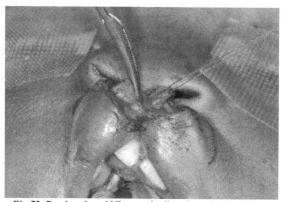

Fig.72 Passing the middle muscle sling through the philtrum

Caudal muscle layer suturing

After having sutured all 6 muscle slings, finish the caudal muscle layer belonging to the red part of the lip. You do this with a vicryl stitch going through the cranial part of red muscle part parallel to and just below the white roll, with the knot on the deep side. Check if the white roll is more-or-less continuous.[225]

Final closure suturing

Subcutaneous Now use, as needed, some vicryl 5-0 subcutaneous sutures to bring the skin into its correct position.

Cutaneous Finish by suturing the skin with catgut 6-0. If you have the opportunity to remove the sutures after 5-7 days, you might prefer to use nylon 6-0.

First, suture the Cupid's bow highest landmarks to their corresponding match (2-9 and 3-14).

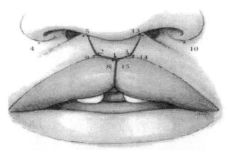

Fig 73Bilateral cleft after complete closure.

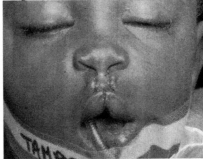

Fig 74.A patient after surgery. Notice the relatively narrow width of the upper lip and the short columella and philtrum

TENNISON TRIANGULAR FLAP TECHNIQUE

This is a direct adaptation of the Tennison flap for unilateral clefts. The procedure for unilateral clefts is done on both sides. This repair results in zigzag scars. The central part of the vermilion margin protrudes in a more normal manner than is achieved with the straight-line repair. Usually, a two-stage procedure is necessary, one side repaired at a time.[225]

MILLARD REPAIR FOR INCOMPLETE CLEFTS

This is an adaptation of the Millard's rotational-advancement method of unilateral cleft lip repair, for use in bilateral cleft cases. In patients with a short prolabium, this procedure moves the prolabium from the nose component into the natural philtrum position of the lip.

155

OTHER TECHNIQUES

Other popular techniques of bilateral cleft lip repair include those of *Bauer et al (1971)*, *Manchester method (1971)*, *Skoog method (1965)*, *Wynn method (1960)*, *Barsky technique (1950 – modification of Veau II operation 1931)*, *primary Abbè flap*, *Mulliken method (1985)*, *Black's method (1985)* and *Noordhoff method (1986)*.

Cleft palate repair

If the anterior palate has not been corrected at the time of the lip repair, it should be done before the premaxilla and maxillary segments are forced together by the action of the repaired lip. This is often done within a few months or weeks after the lip repair, before the child begins to talk.

COMPLICATIONS

1. Wound infection

2. Wound disruption / spreading of scar only supporting tapes should be used in the initial phase. No definitive repair should be attempted until all the induration has subsided.

3. Tilting or retrusion of premaxilla

4. Whistle deformity may be prevented by augmenting the thickness of the prolabium

5. Excessively long lip

6. Collapse of maxillary segments behind the premaxilla

   - this may be prevented or the collapsed segments may be expanded with an acrylic screw or spring plates.

   -

HISTORY OF CLEFT PALATE REPAIR

CLEFT PALATE REPAIR

A cleft palate (palatoschisis) is a fissure in the roof of the oral cavity. It is usually a congenital deformity that leads to abnormal communication between the oral and nasal cavities. Other related classical terms are staphyloschisis (cleft of soft palate) and uranoschisis (cleft of hard palate).[226,227]

HISTORY

Unlike cleft lip surgeries, the techniques for repairing cleft palate have not been mentioned in any of the early literature. All the literature before 1800s mention only the use of prosthetic obturators. *von Graefe (1816) and Roux (1819)*[226,227] successfully closed clefts of the soft palate. *Dieffenbach (1828, 1848)*[226,227] recommended separation of hard palate mucosa from bone as a means of closing the hard palate. *von Langenbeck (1859, 1861)*[226,227] extended these concepts, and described a bipedicled flap procedure. The 19th century further witnessed evolution of the importance of relaxing incisions to reduce the tension of repair. *Veau (1931)*[226,227] converted the bipedicled flaps of von Langenbeck to single pedicled flaps based on greater palatine vessels, and emphasised the need for palatal lengthening. *Wardill (1937) and Kilner (1937) modified Veau's*[226,227] procedure. *Dorrance and Barnsfield (1946)* described the use of a skin graft in the raw palatal surface after the procedure. *Kriens in 1970 and 1975*[227] introduced intravelar veloplasty, which involved releasing of the soft palate muscles from their abnormal bony insertions and resuturing them. The subsequent interest in muscular reconstruction resulted in the development of a double reversing Z-plasty palatoplasty by *Furlow (1980, 1986)*. *Lexan (1908) and Drachter (1914)*[227] first described attempts at bone grafting of the alveolus and palate. Although many surgeons have followed it up, opinion is still divided on the beneficial effects of bone grafting. *Warren (1828)*[227] noted that wide clefts of the hard palate could be narrowed by first closing the soft palate, and he advocated delaying hard palate closure until the ages of 5 to 9. Some centres routinely follow this protocol. Other schools of thought prefer closure of hard and soft palate simultaneously, emphasising the beneficial effects on speech development.[227]

ANATOMY OF THE PALATAL CLEFT

A cleft of secondary palate involves both hard and soft palates from the uvula postreriorly to the junction with the primary palate anteriorly at the incisive foramen. The variation in severity of the palatal clefts reflects the antero-posterior sequence of fusion, and the cleft invariably affects the uvula which is the last portion to fuse.

Deficiency of bony palate varies from a notch in the midline at the posterior border, to a V-shaped defect extending along the whole of the secondary palate. Deficiency of the mucosal tissue and bone is the main characteristic of the cleft hard palate. In the soft palate, the deficiency of mucosal tissue is combined with a shortening of the velar musculature, which has abnormal insertions.

An isolated cleft of the secondary palate does not affect the basic growth mechanism of the upper jaw. A cleft of the primary palate leads to a tendency towards maxillary collapse, but this would be countered by an intact secondary palate. However, if both the parts have clefts, there will be a collapse of maxilla on the affected side.

The major difference in the arrangement of muscles in cleft palate is that those muscles extending towards the central line of the soft palate cannot attach themselves to a fixed point in the raphae of the soft palate, and hence they insert at some substitute points. This prevents them from becoming fully functional.

The muscle bundles of palatoglossus and palatopharyngeus bypass the margin of the cleft soft palate and are inserted along the long axes of the posterior edge of the hard palate. Some bundles may proceed still further forward along the cleft margin of the hard palate, like a cleft muscle.

The atypical muscular arrangements contribute to bony changes, the most common being a large hamulus. The pterygopharyngeal part of palatoglossus and superior constrictor compensates for the loss of function of soft palate and forms a prominent Passavant's ridge. Because of abnormal insertions, the muscles of palate act almost in opposite directions to a non-cleft case, and levator constriction usually results in a widening of the cleft.

GENERAL CONSIDERATIONS

An infant born with a cleft palate deformity inherits many handicaps. Unable to develop intra-oral negative pressure, he cannot suckle and cannot feed in a normal fashion. On swallowing, he expels his feeds through the nose. The open cleft, because of its failure to warm and moisten the inspired air, produces a continuous sore throat. The middle ear becomes secondarily involved with recurrent otitis media. Mastoiditis can be a secondary complication.

In clefts involving alveolus and hard palate, the cleft segments may collapse, and produce malocclusion. Speech is invariably affected due to the mis articulation, hyper/ hyponasality, and nasal escape, which interfere with the intelligibility of individual words and sentences. The hypernasal quality of speech is due to velopharyngeal incompetence.

Counseling is an important aspect of cleft palate management. The person counseling the parents should point out the serious functional deficiencies. He should indicate that each of them would be dealt with at the optimum period of the patient's growth. The parents should not be overwhelmed at the primary interviews but at each step, gradual reassurance and training to deal with the patient should be given.

PROSTHETIC OBTURATION

The prosthetic obturation of the cleft palate deformity has a history of several centuries and even as late as 1940s, the results of surgical repair were often poor, resulting in unfavourable sequelae. Thus, it came to be considered that dental prosthesis with a bulb extension beyond the soft palate (to enable superior constrictor to valve against it) was the ideal treatment modality.

But it is now found that the best speech results with obturation are not as good as fair results achieved with surgery. Furthermore, prosthesis puts great stress on remaining teeth. Today, primary prosthetic closure of cleft palate has no place, except in patients who are poor surgical risks, who are impossible to be intubated and in cases where poor surgery has been followed by scarring, fistulas and poor tissue to work with.

THE GOALS OF SURGERY

The primary goals of cleft palate surgery are

A. construction of an air- and water-tight velopharyngeal valve

- This is an essential requisite for normal speech and normal deglutition. If this primary goal is not achieved, the treatment could be deemed at least a partial failure. Secondary procedures are available to improve the results of primary repair. The three procedures used today for constructing a tight valve are

(i) Closure of palate with reconstruction of the levator

muscle sling

(ii) V-Y retropositioning of the palate

(iii) Simultaneous closure of palate and primary

pharyngeal flap

B. Preservation of hearing

C. Preservation of facial growth

-   Retardation of maxillary growth is thought to be the result of excessive scarring produces by the surgery on the palate. The incidence and severity of maxillary deficiency may be reduced by minimising the periosteal elevation at the time of surgery.

D.   Functional occlusion and aesthetic dentition

-   This goal is achieved by the use of pre-surgical orthopaedics and conventional orthodontic therapy. Orthognathic surgery may have to be performed later in cases of severe secondary deformities.

TIMING OF TREATMENT

While a speech pathologist would prefer to have an intact speech mechanism as soon as possible, the orthodontist would like to have a minimum of scarring until the facial growth is completed. In comparing these two contrasting problems, the trade-off is not often even. Established misarticulation of speech is difficult to treat through speech therapy and can interfere drastically with development such as schooling and social activities. Simple cross-bites can be easily treated orthodontically, and major underdevelopment of maxilla may be treated by orthognathic surgery. All these point favourably towards an early surgical repair of a cleft palate. Another factor favouring early surgery is the establishment of a good feeding mechanism.

It has been traditional to close the palatine cleft at 18 to 24 months of age. Today it has come down to 12 to 18 months. There are many surgeons who prefer an even earlier repair at 3 to 9 months of age.

After *Warren (1828)* had noted that wide clefts of the hard palate could be narrowed by first closing the soft palate, *Schweckendick (1955, 1962)* argued for leaving the hard palate unrepaired to allow for maxillary growth before closing the hard palate. A number of centers still adhere to this philosophy, delaying hard palate closure until the ages of 5 to 9 years, to allow the maxilla to achieve most of its lateral growth.

PRE-SURGICAL ORTHOPAEDICS

McNeil (1954) and later Burstone (1960) advocated early manipulation of alveolar and maxillary segments with the purpose of improving dental arch alignment in the infant. At present, surgeons are divided on the benefits of its use.

SURGICAL TECHNIQUES FOR CLEFT PALATE REPAIRE

The child must be in good health and free from respiratory tract infections. While positioning the patient, the head is extended adequately. General anaesthesia is used with an oral endotracheal tube, taped to the midline of the chin. The operative area may be injected with small amounts of 1:1,00,000 epinephrine. A Dingman mouth-gag is used for maximum exposure. Perioperative antibiotics may be helpful.

VON LANGENBECK OPERATION (1859, 1861)

This is an established procedure that includes the elevation of large muco-periosteal flaps from the hard palate. It is a side-to-side approximation of the cleft margins of both hard and soft palate with detachment of levator muscles from their bony attachments.

The edges of the cleft are incised from the alveolus to the base of the uvula, the sides of which are excised. Relaxing incisions are made from the anterior tonsillar pillar at the lateral edges of the soft palate to pass laterally around the maxillary tuberosity to proceed anteriorly between major palatine vessels and the gingiva, up to approximately the level of the premolar teeth.

The incision is carried through the periosteum, and the mucoperiosteum is lifted widely off the base with a blunt elevator. The lateral incisions are opened widely, using scissors in the posterior aspect. A vomerine mucosal layer may be elevated to provide a two-layer hard palate closure.

On either side of the greater palatine vessels, they are gently stretched out of the canal. The levator muscle is completely freed of its bony attachment.

Closure is achieved in three layers in the soft palate using 4-0 or 5-0 chromic catgut sutures. End-on mattress sutures are preferred in the oral mucosal aspect to prevent inversion of the mucosal edges.

VEAU-WARDILL-KILNER OPERATION (1931, 1937, 1937)

Most palatal repairs that fail to achieve velopharyngeal incompetence do so either because there is insufficient motion in the soft palate or the entire repaired palate is not long enough. In the *Wardill-Kilner modification* of the *Veauoperation*, a V-Y lengthening procedure is done on the tissues of the mucoperiosteum of the hard palate. The rigid mucoperiosteum probably maintains the length that is achieved provided similar amount of lengthening is obtained in the nasal mucosa of the palate.

After incising the cleft margins, a S-shaped incision is made starting along the pterygomandibular raphae, curving around maxillary tuberosity and anteriorly, just as in the *von Langenbeck operation*. However, anteriorly in the canine region, the incision continues at right angles to the apex of the cleft. The flap is elevated at the mucoperiosteum-bony interface, back to the posterior palatine foramen, dissecting and preserving the palatine vessels.

The nasal mucosa is separated from the posterior nasal spine and from superior palatine shelves. Then the lateral pharyngeal wall is freed from the medial pterygoid plate.

The nasal mucosa of either side is sutured together using 5-0 or 4-0 chromic catgut as the first layer of palatal closure. In the soft palate, the muscular and mucosal layers are closed as one. A single suture is placed in the nasal mucosa at the junction of hard and soft palate, incorporating the oral mucosa and muscular layers to obliterate any dead space. The anterior ends of the flaps are sutured to each other and to the triangle of mucoperiosteum over the incisive foramen, thus effecting a V-Y lengthening of the palate.

The V-Y lengthening invariably leaves bare membranous bone exposed in the area from where flaps are taken. These areas usually granulates quickly and epithelize promptly in 2-3 weeks. However, they remain as areas of fibrous scar, and probably are the most likely causes of maxillary growth deficiency and production of dental malocclusion.

FURLOW'S DOUBLE REVERSING Z-PLASTY (1980, 1986)

This is a recent development which attempts to combine the palatal closure with lengthening of soft palate. This operation consists of two Z-plasties, one on the oral mucosa of the soft palate and the other in the reverse orientation on the nasal mucosa of the soft palate.

The levator muscle on one side is included in the posteriorly based oral mucosal flap, and the levator muscle on the opposite side is included in the posteriorly based nasal mucosal flap. The hard palate defect is closed by a vomer flap in one or two layers.

The advantage of this operation is that it lengthens the soft palate within the substance of the soft palate, making it unnecessary to raise large mucoperiosteal flaps from the hard palate with possible retardation of maxillary growth. In addition, the *Furlow operation* reorients the malposition of the levator muscles allowing approximation of the muscles in an overlapped position, and also avoids wide muscular dissection. Moreover, a straight midline incision on the soft palate is avoided. The length and limit of the Z-plasty vary inversely with the width of the cleft.

BONE GRAFTING

Bone grafting of the alveolus has long been a concern in both unilateral and bilateral clefts with alveolar involvement. Studies in early bone grafting in the first year of life by *Pruzansky and Adnis (1964)* show no worthwhile benefits of this procedure. Studies also appeared showing that early bone grafting tended to restrain the maxillary growth rather than supplement it. But recent reports by *Nylen et al, Rosenstein et al* etc. who had continued the use of early bone grafts, show very good results.

Bone grafts in the alveolar cleft not only tend to stabilise the adjacent bony segments but also provide a matrix into which the adjacent permanent teeth can erupt. Without this bone matrix, the teeth usually angle away from the alveolar ridge and erupt in a diagonal fashion. Sources of bone tissue include iliac crest, calvarium, rib and tibia. Cancellous bone chips are preferred over intact blocks.

A protocol popularized by **Abyholm et al (1981)** recommends packing of cancellous bone into the cleft at 9-11 years of age when the adjacent permanent teeth are erupting. The cleft area is opened as a 'trap-door' type of flap and coverage is achieved by these flaps made of gingival tissue. Bonded orthodontic appliances or post-operative retainer plates may be used to ensure best positioning of adjacent teeth and to stabilize the movable segments. **Skoog (1965)** reported the use of maxillary periosteum in a technique called 'bone-less bone grafting' for the closure of the palatal defect.

The technique of bone grafting as mentioned by **Wolfe et al (1983)** is as follows: After preliminary injection with an epinephrine-saline solution, a superiorly based mucogingival triangular flap is elevated, as far as possible into the depth of the alveolar cleft. An incision is made along the edges of the cleft, midway between the palate and the nasal floor. Superiorly based flaps are developed for nasal lining and inferiorly based flaps are reflected caudally for palatal lining. The dissection should extent posteriorly beyond the extent of palatal cleft. The nasal lining is closed with fine catgut or Vicryl sutures. The palatal closure is achieved with larger sutures. Then the bone graft is packed into the entire extent of the cleft, thus providing bone for the nasal floor and palate. Bone is also used to constitute a piriform rim. The previously developed triangular flap is then brought down for anterior alveolar closure without tension. When there has been a poor lip repair, reopening the lip facilitates closure of large alveolar clefts.

POST-OPERATIVE CARE

The patients are observed carefully for 12 hours or more. The airway should be monitored closely. A fingertip pulse oxygen monitor is a helpful guide to post-operative aeration.

Intravenous fluids are given to keep the child hydrated. Full liquids are offered by mouth usually in the afternoon of surgery. The tongue sutures may be removed 24-48 hours after surgery. Bottle with nipples must not be used as undue negative pressure in the suture line can cause disruption.

Arm-cuffs (elbow splints) are used continuously and are maintained for 3 weeks. Soft baby food can be started at third day after surgery. Feedings are followed by water to clear food particles. The diet is continued for three weeks after which normal diet is resumed.

Post-operatively (after discharge), they are seen at three week intervals. Mothers are encouraged to talk to their children and to encourage sucking and using whistles and mouth organs to stimulate velopharyngeal closure. Close monitoring of speech development is necessary. Speech therapy may have to be instituted to correct any speech defects.

COMPLICATIONS

A number of complications may be associated with the correction of cleft palate.

1. Impaired airway –

    - The airway may be impaired during surgery by secretions or bleeding. A nasopharyngeal airway (no.18 or no.20) may be used. A tongue stitch taped to the cheek may be helpful in preventing airway collapse.

2. Bleeding –

    - With the use of vasoconstrictive agents, bleeding is rarely brisk, and is easily controlled by cautery or gauze packing. Ligatures should be reduced to a minimum, but may be done if necessary. Blood replacement should be rarely necessary.

3. Dehiscence –

    - Suturing of the mucoperiosteal flaps under tension invites wound disruption when the patient cries, speaks or eats. Sedation will help to control crying. Disruption due to acute causes may be repaired immediately. If infection has set in, it is better to wait till the acute symptoms subside.

4. Fistulas –

    - This is a frequent complication of cleft palate surgery. One common reason is the failure to incise the epithelium completely at the cleft edges. Oro-nasal fistulas are usually corrected only by secondary procedures.

5.   Nasal speech –

- Persistent nasal speech may be corrected by speech therapy or by secondary pharyngoplasty techniques.

SECONDARY DEFORMITIES OF CLEFT LIP/PALATE REPAIR

Secondary deformities can exist after the repair of cleft lip and palate, and can affect some or all of the previously cleft regions. The degree of the deformities is related to several variables – the severity of the original defect, the method of repair and subsequent healing, the inherent and familial patterns of the patient's craniofacial growth, the effectiveness of orthodontic therapy and adequacy of prosthetic rehabilitation. Secondary deformities of the cleft lip/palate may be classified into

(a)   Lip deformities

(b)   Nose deformities

(c)   Palatal fistula / velopharyngeal incompetence

(d)   Maxillary deficiency or asymmetry[236]

SECONDARY DEFORMITIES OF THE UNILATERAL CLEFT[236]

LIP DEFORMITIES

The secondary lip deformities are of wide variety in type and severity. They include lip scars, long lip (vertical excess), short lip (vertical deficiency), tight lip (horizontal deficiency), muscle abnormalities, vermilion border deformities, deficiency of buccal sulcus etc[236237]

Lip scars

Lip scars are unavoidable. Revision techniques include Z- or W-plasty or wave line excisions. Scar revisions should be designed to correct the specific deformity as it affects the skin, muscle and mucosa. In order to reduce the severity of scar deformity, it is preferable to remove the sutures within 4 days and use adhesive tapes later.[236,237]

Long lip (vertical excess)

Some flap repairs like *Tennison-Randall* and *LeMesurier* can produce this deformity when precise measurements are not subscribed to. It may also occur as a result of excessive rotation of a Millard flap. This condition is corrected by a full-thickness horizontal excision from the superior portion of the lip below the nostril sill so that the resultant scar is placed in a hidden region.[237]

Short lip (vertical deficiency)

A short lip usually presents as a notching of the previously clefted region of the lip. The commonest cause is a vertical scar contracture along a suture line. It may also occur as a result of inadequate rotation of the medial flap. If the deformity is minor, excision of the scar and a Z-plasty placed close to the nasal sill in the shadow of the nostril may be adequate. The Hagedorn-LeMesurier technique may be suitable for cases in which cupid's bow is destroyed.[236,238]

Tight lip (horizontal deficiency)

Sacrifice of excessive tissue during the primary repair produces an in-drawn upper lip, which is stretched across the teeth. Correction of this lip disproportion may require an Abbè flap, which is a 180° transposition of a lower lip flap, inserted into the upper lip. In many cases, maxillary advancement by orthognathic surgery alone restores the upper lip profile more satisfactorily than does an Abbè flap.[236,237,238]

Orbicularis oris abnormalities

These include muscle deficiency, discontinuity or diastasis. Various techniques of muscle dissection and reorientation have been described. In the case of a diastasis, a Z-plasty incorporating the scarred medial and lateral segments may be done.[236]

Vermilion border deficiency

This is the most common secondary deformity. It may be corrected by Z-plasties, V-Y advancements, transposition flaps, free grafts or cross lip flaps.[240]

Deficient buccal sulcus

This frequent problem is managed using V-Y or V-Z advancements.

Nasal deformity

A unilateral cleft lip deformity characteristically involves an asymmetric nose. On the cleft side, the alar base is displaced posteriorly, inferiorly and laterally. The alar cartilage is usually unfolded and may droop down below the level of free edge normal alar cartilage. The nasal spine and columella are displaced towards the non-cleft side. Any of these problems might persist after primary surgery. Usual corrective secondary surgeries include rotation of the cleft lip lobule and external incisions, and alar cartilage mobilisation and suspension.

Proper repair of the unilateral cleft nasal deformity requires unilateral columellar lengthening and repositioning of the lower lateral cartilage. It may be accomplished by wide undermining of the tip and nares as well as the space between the medial crura.[236,244,245]

Maxillary deformities and malocclusion

Maxillary deformities are thought to be the result of associated palatal clefts. These deformities are described and their management discussed in the portion dealing with 'secondary deformities of cleft palate'.[242,243]

SECONDARY DEFORMITIES OF THE BILATERAL CLEFT

As with the case of unilateral lefts, the bilateral cleft lip cases also have their share of residual deformities requiring secondary treatment. They may be deformities of lip, nose and/or premaxilla.[240,241,242]

Lip deformities

The most common lip deformities include

    A. V-shaped whistle deformity in the midpoint of the lip

    B. short prolabium

    C. wide prolabium

    D. asymmetric vermilion

    E. immobile prolabium

    F. inadequate orbicularis oris repair

    G. deficient gingivo-buccal sulcus

    H. tight upper lip

    I. long upper lip

The thin central vermilion (whistle deformity) is more commonly seen after the Manchester type of repair. Bilateral V-Y advancement or bilateral vermilion island flaps may be used for the correction of the whistle deformity. If the deficiency of the gingivo-buccal sulcus is caused by an adhesion, the adhesion may be split, and the defect closed in the form of an Z-plasty. Most other problems are corrected by techniques similar to those used for unilateral cleft cases.[240,241,242]

Nose deformity

The predominant deformity of bilateral cleft nose is that of a short columella. The nose deformity is usually symmetric, with a short or absent columella and inferiorly displaced medial crura of alar cartilages. Bifid nasal tip and lateral displacement of alar bases on the retruded maxilla are also characteristic. Various techniques of columellar lengthening, cartilage dissection and alar repositioning have been described by many authors. If the tissue is very deficient in the columella, length may be gained with a V-Y advancement of the mid-vertical portion of the prolabium in continuity with the columella. An alternative is the use of forked flaps. Conchal cartilage grafts may be helpful to obtain adequate tip projection.[244,245]

SECONDARY DEFORMITIES OF CLEFT PALATE

The most important secondary deformities of palatal clefts are persistent nasal speech, palatal fistulas and velopharyngeal incompetence, apart from maxillary deformities and dental malocclusion.[236]

Palatal fistula

The most common defect in the hard palate after repair is a fistula. It may be located anterior or posterior to the incisive foramen, and are more frequent in cases of combined clefts of primary and secondary palates. True fistulas are caused by infection, haematoma formation between the oral and nasal layers, excess tension on the repair, flap necrosis, inadequate attachment of the oral to the nasal layer, and a technically insecure anterior closure.[243]

Palatal fistulas may present as asymptomatic holes, or may cause such symptoms as speech problems and difficulties with dental hygiene. Large defects that affect speech or allow escape of fluid or food particles through the nose, should be closed early. When the fistula is small, closure can be delayed or not performed at all. Closure of defects between the oral cavity and the nasal and maxillary sinus cavities should always be two-layered, by turning medial and lateral flaps from the cleft margin to form the nasal floor and rotating one or two

Veau flaps medially with a buccal or preferably gingival flap for oral closure. When the alveolar fistula is closed, the alveolar defect should be bone grafted.[243]

Another option is an anteriorly or posteriorly based tongue flaps. Although infrequently necessary, the use of an obturator is an alternative solution in defects that cannot be closed by local tissue because of size or because of patient preference.[243]

Velopharyngeal incompetence

Velopharyngeal incompetence (VPI) is the condition where the patient is not able to close the velopharyngeal sphincter, which separates oropharynx from nasopharynx, completely. It may be due to a structural defect or physiologic dysfunction. The shortness of palate following surgery is attributed to the original inadequacy of the palatal tissue rather than to the inadequacies of surgery. The main characteristic of VPI is the hypernasal quality of speech, which is due to the increase in the amount of air passing through the nose, thus adding the resonance of the nasal passages and paranasal sinuses in the production of sounds.[236]

The procedures available for the correction of VPI are

1.   Palatal lengthening procedures

2.   Pharyngeal flaps

3.   Augmentation of the posterior pharyngeal wall

4.   reconstruction of velopharyngeal sphincter

REFERENCES

1. .Peterson,Ellis,hupp,Tucker contemporary oral and maxillofacial surgery ,5th ed St Louis M.S. by 2003

2. The origin of term "Harelip" by J.DOUGLAS NOLL, Ph.D. lafeyette,Indiana 47907.

3. .Tretment of cleft lip and palate during the Revolutionary War ; bicentennial Reflection (Blair O. Rogers ,M.D.) New York City ,New York

4. Cleft lip Cleft Palate their Manegment Dr.Shriprakash Kumar B.D.S. DHLS,DMR .DED JMISM INDRESH NAGAR ,PATANA

5. .Converse Chapter 38 John Morquis Converse,V.Michel Hogasn,Josheph G Maccarty

6. GORLIN R.J. CERVENKA J, AND PROZANASKY S : Facial clefting and its syndrome , birth defects : Original article series , 1971; 7;3- 49

7. .The dental clinics of North America :Genetics, 1975; 19(1)..

8. FOGH ANDERSON P: Fistula Labii inferiors congenital, Saertryle al Tandl aegebladet, 1943; 47: 411-417

9. . CERVENKA J, GORLIN R.J. AND ANDERSON V.E: The syndrome of pits of the lower lip and cleft lip and/or palate , Genetic considerations: Amer. J. Hum. Genet, 1967; 19:446-432.

10..ALEXANDRE REZENDE VIEIRA, IEDA MARIA ORIOLE: Journal of Dentistry for children: July August 2001; 272-279.

11..HOLKOVA R, MOLNAROVA A, NEMICK. BROZMAN M, FABRY J, HARAKOVA E.: Relation between toxoplasmosis and orofacial clefts in children: Bartisl lek listy, 1974; 95(2) :64-7.

12..NATSUME M, KAWAI T, OGI M, YOSHIDA W: Maternal risk factors in cleft lip and palate, case control study : Br. J. Oral maxillofac. Surg., 2000; 38(1) 23-5.

13..SHAW G.M., WASSEMAN CR, LAMMER E.J. , O'MALLEY, MURRY J.C., BASANT AM, TOLAROVA MM : Orofacial clefts, parental cigarette smoking and transforming growth factor – alpha gene variants: Am J. Human Genet 1996 Mar; 58(3):551-61.

14..NAGATO NATSUME, FUMIHIKO SATO, KOUJI HARA, TSUYOSHI KAWAI, NOBUMI OGI: Description of Japanese twins with cleft lip, left palate or both: Oral Surg. Oral Med, Oral Pathol, Oral Radial Endod. 2000; 89, 6-8.

15..FRASER F.C : The genetics of clefts lips and palate: Am. J. Hum. Genet.1970; 22; 336.

16..JOSEPH G. MC CARTHY : Cleft lip and Craniofacial Anomalies, Plastic surgery Vol.4

17..ALYSWORTH A.S: Genetic considerations in cleft lip and palate :Clin. Plan. Surg.1985; 12:533.

18..CHUNG K.S., KAU M.S: Racial difference in cephalometric measurements and incidence of cleft lip with and without cleft palate: J.Cranifac Dev Biol 1985;(5)4:341-9.

19..WOOLF C.M: Paternal age affect on cleft lip and palate : Am. J, Hum Genet, 1963; 15:389.

20..FRASER G.R. AND CALNAN J.S: Cleft lip and palate:Seasonal incidence, birth weight, birth rank, sex site associated malformation and parental age: Arch Die child,1961; 36: 420.

21..LAENDER J.M.; TANNIR; H; AND SADLER; J.H: Serotonin and morphogensis. Sites of serotonin uptake and binding protein immunoractivity in the mid gestation mouse embryo: Development, 1998; 102; 702.

22..PATTERSON S.B., AND MINKOFF R: Morphometric and audio-radiographic analysis of frontonasal development in the chick.: Anat. Rec.1985; 212: 90.

23..GAARE J.D. AND LANGMAN J: Fusion of nasal swelling in the mouse embryo. Surface coat and intrinsic contact: Am . J. Anat.1977; 150:461.

24..SMILEY G AND VANIK, R.J AND DIXON A.D: Width of the craniofacial complexes during formation of the secondary palate: Cleft Palate J,1971; 8:371.

25..DAVIDSON J.G., FRASER F.C. AND SCHLAGER G: A maternal effect on the frequency of spontaneous cleft lip in the A/J mouse: Teratology, 1969; 2: 371.

26..BIDDLE F.G. AND FRASER FC: Major gene determination of liability to spontaneous cleft lip in the mouse: J. Craniofacial Genetic Dev.Biol. 1986; 2:67.

27..LANDAUER W.J. SOPHER D: Succinate glycerophosphate and ascorbate as sources of cellular energy and as antiteratogens: J. Embryol. Exp. Morphol, 1970; 24: 187.

28..KHOURY M.J., WEINSTEIN A. PANNY S., HOTTZMAN N.A., LINDSAY P.K: Maternal cigarette smoking and oral clefts; a population based study: Am. J. Public Health , 1987; 77: 623.

29..SULIK K.K., JOHNSTON M.C., AMBORSE L.J AND DROGAN D: Phenytoin (Dilantin) induced cleft lip and palate in A/J mice:A scanning and transmission electron microscopic study: Anat. Rec.,1979; 195; 243.

30..ASLING C.W: Congenital defects of the face and palate following maternal deficiency of pteroyl glutomic acid: In Pruzansky , S (Ed). Congenital anomalies of the face and associated structures, Springfield IL, Charles C, Thomas 1961.

31..LAURENCE K.M: Causes of neural tube malformation and through prevention by dietary improvement and pre-conceptional supplementation with folic acid and multivitamins: In Briggs M. (Ed). Recent Vitamin research Boca Raten, FL, CRC, 1984.

32.BIGGS, R.M: Vitamin supplementation as a possible factor in the incidence of cleft lip, palate deformities in humans: Clin. Plast.Surg., 1976; 3; 647.

33. ROSS, C.B., AND JOHNSTEN, M.C: Cleft Lip and palate: Baltimore, Williams and Wilkins company, 1972.

34. BURDI, A.R AND SILVEY R.G: Sexual differences in closure of human palatal shelves : Cleft Palate J,1969; 6:1.

35. .GRABER T.M: The congenital cleft palate deformity: J. Am. Dent. Assoc.1954; 48:375.

36. .JOLLEYS A : A review of the results of operations on cleft palates with references to maxillary growth and speech function: Br. J. Plast. Surg., 1954; 7:229.

37. DAHL E: Craniofacial morphology in congenital clefts of the lip and palate: Acta odontal scand., 1970; 29 (57): 11.

38. .BISHARA S.E. AND IVORSON W.W: Cephalometric comparisons on the cranial base and face in individuals with isolated clefts of the palate : Cleft Palate Journal , 1974; 11: 162.

39. SMAHEL, Z, AND BREJCHA M : Differences in craniofacial morphology between complete and incomplete unilateral cleft lip and palate in adults: Cleft Palate J, 1983; 20:113.

40. .ROSS R.B: Treatment various affecting facial growth n complete unilateral cleft lip and palate: Part I. Cleft Palate J., 1987; 24:5.

41. .ROSS R.B. AND JOHNSTON M.C: Cleft Lip and palate: Baltimore,Williams and Wilkins company 1972.

42. .NARULA J AND ROSS R.B: Facial growth in children with complete bilateral cleft lip and palate: Cleft Palate J,1970; 7: 239.

43. .ROSS R.B: The clinical implications of facial growth in cleft lip and palate: Cleft palate J., 1970; 7:37.

44. .ROSS R.B: Treatment variables affecting facial growth in complete unilateral cleft lip palate, Part.3, Alveolar repair and bone grafting: Cleft palate J,1987; 24: 33.

45..SHWECKENDICK W: Primary veloplasty :long term results without maxillary deformity. A twenty five year report: Cleft Palate J, 1978; 15: 268.

46..HOLZ, M.M. GNOINSKI, W.M., NUSSBAUMER, H AND KISTLER, E: Early maxillary orthopedics in CLP cases ; guidelines for surgery: Cleft Palate J, 1978; 15: 405

47..BHJDORP P AND EGYEDI P : The influence of age at operation for cleft on the development of the jaws: J. Maxillofacial surgery, 1984; 12:193.

48..ROSS R.B: Treatment variables affecting facial growth in complete unilateral cleft lip palate. Part 5 Timing of cleft palate repair: Cleft palate J, 1987; 24 : 54.

49..ROSS R.B: Treatment variables affecting facial growth in complete unilateral cleft palate.Part 6, Technique of cleft palate repair: Cleft Palate J, 1987; 24: 64.

50..TONDURY G: On the mechanisms of cleft formation: In Pruzansky S. (Ed). Congenital anomalies of the face and associated structures. Srungfeild, IL, Charles Thomas, 1961, 85-101.

51.. Bohn A: Dental anomalies in harelip and cleft palate: Acta Odontal Scand, 1963; 21(suppl):38.

52. RATNA R: The development of the permanent teeth in children with complete cleft lip and palate :Proc. Finn Dent. Soc, 1971; 67: 350-355.

53. ABDULLA A., SADOWSKY C., BEGOOE EA : Deciduous tooth dimensions in cleft lip and palate: Cleft Palate J. 1984;21:301-307.

54..GRAHNEN H, GRANATH L-E : Numerical variations in primary dentiton and their correlation with the permanent dentition: Odont. Rev. 1961;12:348-357.

55..DIXON DA: Defects of structure and formation of teeth in persons with cleft palate and the effect or reparative surgery on the dental tissues: Oral Surg. 1968:25:435-446.

56..RAVN J. J : Aplasia,Supernumerary teeth and fused teeth in the primary dentition. An epidemiologic study: Scand J Dent. Res. 1971:791-6.

57....LAVELLE CL B: A note on the variation in the timing of deciduous tooth eruption: J. Dent. 1975;3:267-270.

58..BAGHDADY VS. CHOSE LJ: Eruption time of primary teeth in Iraqi children: Community Dent. Oral Epidemiol. 1981;9:245-246

59..LAUZIER C. DEMIRJAIAN A.L : L' emergence des dents primaries chez l'enfant candadien-francais: Union Med Can. 1981; 110:1061-1064.

60..LUNT RC, LAW DB : A review of the chronology of eruption of deciduous teeth: J Am Dent. Assoc. 1974b; 89:872-879.

61..NYSTROM M, KILPINEN E: KLEEMOLA KUJALA E: A radio-graphic study of the formation of some teeth from 0.5 to 3.0 years of age: Proc. Finn Dent. Soc. 1977;73:167-172.

62..RANTA R, STEGARS T, RINTALA A: Correlations of hypodontia in children with isolated cleft palate: Cleft Palate J. 1983; 20, 163-165.

63..FOSTER TD, LAVELLE CL B: The size of the dentition in complete cleft lip and palate: Cleft Palate J. 1971;8:177-184.

64..ADAMS MS, NISWANDER, JD: Developmental "Noise" and a congenital malformation: Genet Res. 1967:10:313-317.

65..SOFAER JA : Human tooth size asymmetry in cleft lip with or without cleft palate: Arch Oral Biol. 1979;24:141-146.

66.. HUNTER WS, DIJKMAN DF: The timing of height and weight deficits in twins discordant for cleft lip and/or palate: Cleft Palate J. 1977:14:158-166

67. RANTA R: Comparison of tooth formation in noncleft and cleft affected children with and without hypodontia: ASDC J Dent. Child. 1982;49:197-199.

68. .RANTA R: Associations of some variables of tooth formation in children with isolated cleft palate: Scand J Dent. Res. 1984;92:492-502.

69. .GARN SM, LEWIS AB, POLACHECK DL: Interrelations in dental development. I. Interrelationships within the dentition: J Dent. Res. 1960;39:1049-1055.

70. LYSELL L. MAGNUSSON B. THILANDER B : Time and order of eruption of the primary teeth: Odont. Rev. 1092; 13:217.

71. .KENT RL JR., REED RB, MORES CFA : Associations in emergence age among permanent teeth: Am J.Phys Anth. Ropol. 1978;48:131-142.

72. .GARN SM, SMITH BH: Developmental communalities in tooth emergence timing: J Dent. Res. 1980b;59: 1178.

73. .LYSELL L, MAGNUSSON B, THILANDER B: Relations between the times of eruption of primary and permanent teeth: Acta Odontol Scand. 1969:27:271-281.

74. .TARANGER J, LICHTENSTEIN H, SVENNBERG.REDEGREN I: Dental development from birth to 16 years: Acta Pediatr Scand. 1976; (suppl. 258):83-97.

75. .NYSTROM M: Development of the deciduous dentition in a series of Finnish children: Proc. Finn Dent. Soc. 1977; 73:155-166.

76. .BAILIT HL, NISWANDER JD, MACLEAN C: The relationship among several prenatal factors and variations in the permanent dentition in Japanese Children: Growth 1968b:32:331-345.

77. .BAILIT HL, SUNG B: Maternal effects on the developing dentition: Arch Oral Biol.1968:13:155-161.

78. .GARN SM : Osborne RH, McCabe KD : The effect of prenatal factors on crown dimensions: Am J Phys Anthropol. 1979;51:665-678.

79. .GARN SM, OBSORNE RH : ALVESALO L, HOROWITZ SL: Material and gestational influences on deciduous and permanent tooth size: J of Dent Res.1980a;59:142-143

80. .WEYERS H: Der Durchbruch der Milchzahne. Munchen, Germany :Carl Hanser Verlag; 1968, : J. Dent. Res. 1980a;59:142-143

81. .GOLDEN NL. TAKIEDDINE F, HIRSCH VJ : Teething age in prematurely born infants: Am J. Dis child. 1981;135:903-904.

82. KURT. W. BUTOW: Treatment of facial cleft deformities.An illustrated guide,1996.

83. GISELE DA SILVA DALBEN, BEATRIZ COSTA, MARCIA RIBEIRO,GOMIDE, LUCIMARA TEIXEIRA DAS NEVES: Dental anaesthetic procedures for cleft lip and palate patients: J Clin Pediatr Dent 2000; 24(3):153-157.

84. .MULLEROVA Z, SMAHEL Z: Effects of primary osteoplasty on facial growth in unilateral cleft lip and palate after ten years of follow-up: Acta Chir Plast. 1989;31(3):181-91

85. SMAHEL Z: Effects of certain therapeutic factors on facial development in isolated cleft palate: Acta Chir Plast. 1989;31(1):35-47.

86. ENEMARK H, BOLUND S, JORGENSEN I: Evaluation of unilateral cleft lip and palate treatment: long term results: Cleft Palate J.1990Oct;27(4):354-61.

87. SMAHEL Z, HORAK I: Effects of soft tissue and osseous bridge on facial configuration in adults with unilateral cleft lip and palate: Acta Chir Plast. 1993;35(3-4):165-72.

88. .TROTMAN CA, ROSS RB: Craniofacial growth in bilateral cleft lip and palate: ages six years to adulthood: Cleft Palate Craniofac J. 1993 May;3 0(3):261-73

89. MOLSTED K, DAHL E, BRATTSTROM V, MCWILLIAM J, SEMB G: A six-center international study of treatment outcome in patients with clefts of the lip and palate: evaluation of maxillary asymmetry: Cleft Palate Craniofac J. 1993 Jan;30(1):22-8.

90. SMAHEL Z: Treatment effects on facial development in patients with unilateral cleft lip and palate: Cleft Palate Craniofac J. 1994 Nov;31(6):437-45.

91. SMAHEL Z, MULLEROVA Z: Facial growth and development in unilateral cleft lip and palate during the period of puberty: comparison of the development after periosteoplasty and after primary bone grafting: Cleft Palate Craniofac J. 1994 Mar;31(2):106-15.

92. .SMAHEL Z, MULLEROVA Z: Facial growth and development in unilateral cleft lip and palate from the time of palatoplasty to the onset of puberty: a longitudinal study: J Craniofac Genet Dev Biol. 1995 Apr-Jun;15(2):72-80.

93. SMAHEL Z, MULLEROVA Z: Craniofacial growth and development in unilateral cleft lip and palate.Clinical Implications (a review): Acta Chir Plast. 1995;37(1):29-32.

94. SMAHEL Z, MULLEROVA Z, HORAK I: Facial development in unilateral cleft lip and palate prior to the eruption of permanent incisors after primary bone grafting and periosteal flap surgery: Acta Chir Plast. 1996;38(1):30-6.

95. SMAHEL Z, MULLEROVA Z: Postpubertal growth and development of the face in unilateral cleft lip and palate as compared to the pubertal period: a longitudinal study: J Craniofac Genet Dev Biol. 1996 Jul-Sep;16(3):182-92.

96. SAMESHIMA GT, BANH DS, SMAHEL Z, MELNICK M: Facial growth after primary periosteoplasty versus primary bone grafting in unilateral cleft lip and palate: Cleft Palate Craniofac J. 1996 Jul;33(4):300-5.

97. CAPELOZZA FILHO L, NORMANDO AD, DA SILVA FILHO OG: Isolated influences of lip and palate surgery on facial growth. Comparison

of operated and unoperated male adults with UCLP: Cleft Palate Craniofac J. 1996 Jan;33(1):51-6.

98.. CASAL C, RIVERA A, RUBIO G, SENTIS-VILALTA J, ALONSO A, GAY-ESCODA C: Examination of craniofacial morphology in 10-month to 5-year-old children with cleft lip and palate: Cleft Palate Craniofac J. 1997 Nov;34(6):490-7.

99. SMAHEL Z, MULLEROVA Z, NEJEDLY A, HORAK I: Changes in craniofacial development due to modifications of the treatment of unilateral cleft lip and palate: Cleft Palate Craniofac J. 1998 May;35(3):240-7.

100. SMAHEL Z, MULLEROVA Z, NEJEDLY A: Effect of primary repositioning of the nasal septum on facial growth in unilateral claft lip and palate : Cleft Palate Craniofac J.1999 Jul;36(4):310-3

101. SCHULTES G, GAGGL A, KARCHER H: A comparison of growth impairment and orthodontic results in adult patients with clefts of palate and unilateral clefts of lip, palate and alveolus: Br J Oral Maxillofac Surg. 2000 Feb;38(1):26-32.

102. PELTOMAKI T, VENDITTELLI BL, GRAYSON BH, CUTTING CB, BRECHT LE: Associations between severity of clefting and maxillary growth in patients with unilateral cleft lip and palate treated with infant orthopedics: Cleft Palate Craniofac J. 2001 Nov;38(6):582-6.

103. ZUO H, SHI B, DENG D, ZHENG G, BAI D: Inhibitive effects of lip repair on maxillary growth in patients with complete unilateral cleft lip and palate: Hua Xi Kou Qiang Yi Xue Za Zhi. 2001 Aug;19(4):229-31

104. FANG B, ZHAO Y: Effects of unilateral cleft lip and palate prosthesis on the development of maxillary and facial soft tissue: Hua Xi Kou Qiang Yi Xue Za Zhi. 2001 Aug;19(4):225-8.

105. DIBIASE AT, DIBIASE DD, HAY NJ, SOMMERLAD BC: The relationship between arch dimensions and the 5-year index in the primary dentition of patients with complete UCLP: Cleft Palate Craniofac J. 2002; 39(6):635-40.

106. KONST EM, RIETVELD T, PETERS HF, PRAHL-ANDERSEN B: Phonological development of toddlers with unilateral cleft lip and palate who were treated with and without infant orthopedics: a randomized clinical trial: Cleft Palate Craniofac J. 2003 Jan;40(1):32-9.

107. GAGGL A, FEICHTINGER M, SCHULTES G, SANTLER G, PICHLMAIER M, MOSSBOCK R, KARCHER H: Cephalometric and occlusal outcome in adults with unilateral cleft lip, palate, and alveolus after two different surgical techniques: Cleft Palate Craniofac J. 2003 May;40(3):249-55.

108. ROSENSTEIN SW, GRASSESCHI M, DADO DV: A long-term retrospective outcome assessment of facial growth, secondary surgical need, and maxillary lateral incisor status in a surgical-orthodontic protocol for complete clefts: Plast Reconstr Surg. 2003 Jan;111(1):1-13; discussion 14-6.

108..Wyszynski, D.F., Beaty, T.H. and Maestri, N.E. (1996) Genetics of nonsyndromic oral clefts revisited. Cleft Palate-Cranio. J., 33, 406–417.

109..Fraser, FC. (1970) The genetics of cleft lip and cleft palate. Am. J. Hum. Genet.,22, 336–352.MedlineW

110..Mitchell, L.E. and Risch, N. (1992) Mode of inheritance of nonsyndromic cleft lip with or without cleft palate: a reanalysis. Am. J. Hum. Genet., 51, 323–332.

111..Wyszynski, D.F. and Beaty, T.H. (1996) Review of the role of potential teratogens in the origin of human nonsyndromic oral clefts. Teratology, 53, 309–317.

112..Wilkie, A.O. and Morriss-Kay, G.M. (2001) Genetics of craniofacial development and malformation. Nat. Rev. Genet., 2, 458–468.

113. .Marazita, M.L., Goldstein, A.M., Smalley, S.L. and Spence, M.A. (1986) Cleft lip with or without cleft palate: reanalysis of a three-generation family study from England. Genet.Epidemiol., 3, 335–342.

114. .Farrall, M. and Holder, S. (1992) Familial recurrence-pattern analysis of cleft lip with or without cleft palate. Am. J. Hum. Genet., 50, 270–277.

115. .Schliekelman, P. and Slatkin, M. (2002) Multiplex relative risk and estimation of the number of loci underlying an inherited disease. Am. J. Hum. Genet., 71, 1369–1385.

116. .Moore, K.L. (1988) The Developing Human, 3rd edn. WB Saunders, Philadelphia, PA, pp. 197–213.

117. .Mo, R., Freer, A.M., Zinyk, D.L., Crackower, M.A., Michaud, J., Heng, H.H., Chik, K.W., Shi, X.M., Tsui, L.C., Cheng, S.H. *et al.* (1997) Specific and redundant functions of *Gli2* and *Gli3* zinc finger genes in skeletal patterning and development.Development, 124, 113–123.

118. .Sanford, L.P., Ormsby, I., Gittenberger-de Groot, A.C., Sariola, H., Friedman, R., Boivin, G.P., Cardell, E.L. and Doetschman, T. (1997) TGFB2 knockout mice have multiple developmental defects are non-overlapping with otherTGFBknockoutphenotypes. Development, 124, 2659–2670.

119. .Rijli, F.M., Mark, M., Lakkaraju, S., Dierich, A., Dolle, P. and Chambon, P. (1993) A homeotic transformation is generated in the rostral branchial region of the head by disruption of Hoxa-2, which acts as a selector gene. Cell, 75, 1333–1349.

120. .Satokata, I. and Maas, R. (1994) *Msx1* deficient mice exhibit cleft palate and abnormalities of craniofacial and tooth development. Nat. Genet., 6, 348–355.

121. .Zhao, Y., Guo, Y.J., Tomac, A.C., Taylor, N.R., Grinberg, A., Lee, E.J., Huang, S. and Westphal, H. (1999) Isolated cleft palate in mice with a

targeted mutation of the LIM homeobox gene Lhx8. Proc. Natl Acad. Sci. USA, 96, 15002–15006.

122. .Ferguson,M.W.(1988)Palatedevelopment. Development, 103 (suppl.), 41–60.

123. .Morris-Wiman, J. and Brinkley, L. (1992) An extracellular matrix infrastructure provides support for murine secondary palatal shelf remodelling. Anat. Rec., 234,575–586.

124. .Peters, H., Neubuser, A., Kratochwil, K. and Balling, R. (1998) Pax9-deficient mice lack pharyngeal pouch derivatives and teeth and exhibit craniofacia and limb abnormalities. Genes Dev., 12, 2735–2747.

125. .Kaartinen, V., Cui, X., Heisterkamp, N., Groffen, J. and Shuler, C.F. (1997) Transforming growth factor-B3 regulates transdifferentiation of medial edge epithelium during palatal fusion and associated degradation of the basement membrane. Dev. Dyn., 209, 255–260.

126. .Martinez-Alvarez, C., Tudela, C., Perez-Miguelsanz, J., O'Kane, S., Puerta, J. and Ferguson, M.W. (2000) Medial edge epithelial cell fate during palatal fusion.Dev. Biol., 220, 343–357.

127. .Bitgood, M.J. and McMahon, A.P. (1995) *Hedgehog* and *Bmp* genes are coexpressed at many diverse sites of cell-cell interaction in the mouse embryo. Dev. Biol., 172, 126–138.

128. .Zhang, Z., Song, Y., Zhao, X., Zhang, X., Fermin, C. and Chen, Y. (2002) Rescue of cleft palate in *Msx1*-deficient mice by transgenic *Bmp4* reveals a network of BMP and Shh signaling in the regulation of mammalian palatogenesis. Development, 129,4135–4146.

129. .Dixon, M.J., Carette, M.J., Moser, B.B. and Ferguson, M.W. (1993) Differentiation of isolated murine embryonic palatal epithelium in culture: exogenous transforming growth factor alpha modulates matrix biosynthesis in defined experimental conditions. In Vitro Cell Dev. Biol., 29A, 51–61.

130. .Ferguson, M.W. and Honig, L.S. (1984) Epithelial-mesenchymal interactions during vertebrate palatogenesis. Curr.Top. Dev. Biol., 19, 137–164.

131. .Richman, J.M. and Lee, S.-H. (2003) About face: signals and genes controlling jaw patterning and identity in vertebrates. BioEssays, 25, 554–568.

132. .Greene, R.M., Nugent, P., Mukhopadhyay, P., Warner, D.R. and Pisano, M.M. (2003) Intracellular dynamics of Smad-mediated TGFβ signalling. J. Cell. Physiol.,197, 261–271.

133. .Fitzpatrick, D.R., Denhez, F., Kondaiah, P. and Akhurst, R.J. (1990) Differential expression of TGF beta isoforms in murine palatogenesis. Development, 109, 585–595.

134. .Proetzel, G., Pawlowski, S.A., Wiles, M.V., Yin, M., Boivin, G.P., Howles, P.N., Ding, J., Ferguson, M.W.J. and Doetschman, T. (1995) Transforming growth factor-β3 is required for secondary palate fusion. Nat. Genet., 11, 409–414.

135. .Kaartinen, V., Voncken, J.W., Shule, C., Warburton, D., Bu, D., Heisterkamp, N. and Groffen, J. (1995) Abnormal lung development and cleft palate in mice lacking TGFB3 indicates defects of epithelial-mesenchymal interaction. Nat. Genet., 11,415–421.

136. .Taya, Y., O'Kane, S. and Ferguson, M.W. (1999) Pathogenesis of cleft palate in TGF-beta3 knockout mice. Development, 126, 3869–3879.

137. .Martinez-Alvarez, C., Bonelli, R., Tudela, C., Gato, A., Mena, J., O'Kane, S. and Ferguson, M.W. (2000) Bulging medial edge epithelial cells and palatal fusion. Int. J. Dev. Biol., 44, 331–335.

138. .Gato, A., Martinez, M.L., Tudela, C., Alonso, I., Moro, J.A., Formoso, M.A., Ferguson, M.W. and Martinez-Alvarez, C. (2002) TGF-beta(3)-induced chondroitin sulphate proteoglycan mediates palatal shelf adhesion. Dev. Biol., 250, 393–405.

139. .Brunet, C.L., Sharpe, P.M. and Ferguson, M.W. (1995) Inhibition of TGF-beta 3 (but not TGF-beta 1 or TGF-beta 2) activity prevents normal mouse embryonic palate fusion. Int. J. Dev. Biol., 39, 345–355.

140. .Blavier, L., Lazaryev, A., Groffen, J., Heisterkamp, N., DeClerck, Y.A. and Kaartinen, V. (2001) TGF-beta3-induced palatogenesis requires matrix metalloproteinases. Mol. Biol. Cell., 12, 1457–1466.

141. .Prescott, N.J., Lees, M.M., Winter, R.M. and Malcolm, S. (2000) Identification of susceptibility loci for nonsyndromic cleft lip with or without cleft palate in a two stage genome scan of affected sib-pairs. Hum. Genet., 106, 345–350.

142. .Marazita, M.L., Field, L.L., Cooper, M.E., Tobias, R., Maher, B.S., Peanchitlertkajorn, S. and Liu, Y.E. (2002) Genome scan for loci involved in cleft lip with or without cleft palate, in Chinese multiplex families. Am. J. Hum. Genet., 71,349–364.

143. .Zeiger, J.S., Hetmanski, J.B., Beaty, T.H., VanderKolk, C.A., Wyszynski, D.F., Bailey-Wilson, J.E., De Luna, R.O., Perandones, C., Tolarova, M.M., Mosby, T. *et al.*(2003) Evidence for linkage of nonsyndromic cleft lip with or without cleft palate to a region on chromosome 2. Eur. J. Hum. Genet., 11, 835–839.

144. .Wyszynski, D.F., Albacha-Hejazi, H., Aldirani, M., Hammod, M., Shkair, H., Karam, A., Alashkar, J., Holmes, T.N., Pugh, E.W., Doheny, K.F. *et al.* (2003) A genome-wide scan for loci predisposing to non-syndromic cleft lip with or without cleft palate in two large Syrian families. Am. J. Med. Genet., 123A, 140–147.

145. .Marazita, M.L., Murray, J.M., Cooper, M., Bailey-Wilson, T.J., Albacha-Hejazi, H., Lidral, A., Moreno, L., Arcos-Bargos, M. and Beaty, T. (2003) Meta-analysis of 11 genome scans for cleft lip with or without cleft palate. Am. J. Hum. Genet., 73,A79.

146. .Vieira, A.R. and Orioli, I.M. (2001) Candidate genes for nonsyndromic cleft lip and palate. ASDCJ Dent. Child., 68, 272–279.

147. .Lowry, R.B. (1970) Sex linked cleft palate in a British Columbian Indian family.Pediatrics; 46, 123–128.

148. .Rushton, A.R. (1979) Sex linked inheritance of cleft palate. Hum. Genet., 48, 179–181.

149. Rollnick, B.R. and Kaye, C.I. (1986) Mendelian inheritance of isolated nonsyndromic cleft palate. Am. J. Med. Genet., 24, 465–473.

150. .Bixler, D. (1987) Letter to the editor: X-linked cleft palate. Am. J. Med. Genet., 28,503–505.

151. .Hall, B.D. (1987) Letter to the editor: A further X-linked isolated nonsyndromic cleft palate family with a nonexpressing obligate affected male. Am. J. Med. Genet., 26,239–240.

152. .Moore, G.E., Ivens, A., Chambers, J., Farrall, M., Williamson, R., Bjornsson, A., Arnason, A. and Jensson, O. (1987) Linkage of an X-chromosome cleft palate gene.Nature, 326, 91–92.

153. .Stanier, P., Forbes, S.A., Arnason, A., Bjornsson, A., Sveinbjornsdottir, E., Williamson, R. and Moore, G.E. (1993) The localisation of a gene causing X-linked cleft palate and ankyloglossia (CPX) in an Icelandic kindred is between DXS326 and DXYS1X. Genomics, 17, 549–555.

154. .Bjornsson, A., Arnason, A. and Tippet, P. (1989) X-linked midline defect in an Icelandic family. Cleft Palate J., 26, 3–8.

155. .Gorski, S.M., Adams, K.J., Birch, P.H., Friedman, J.M. and Goodfellow, P.J. (1992) The gene responsible for X-linked cleft palate (CPX) in a British Columbian native kindred is localized between *PGK1* and DXYS1. Am. J. Hum. Genet., 50, 1129–1136.

156. .Marçano, A.C.B., Ming, J.E., Du, Y.Z., George, R.A., Ryan, S.G., Richieri-Costa, A. and Muenke, M. (2000) X-linked cleft palate and ankyloglossia: refinement of the minimal critical region in Xq21.3. Am. J. Hum. Genet., 67, A1802.

157. .Braybrook, C., Doudney, K., Marçano, A.C.B., Arnason, A., Bjornsson, A., Patton, M.A., Goodfellow, P.J., Moore, G.E. and Stanier, P. (2001) The T-box transcription factor gene *TBX22* is mutated in X-linked cleft palate and ankyloglossia. Nat. Genet., 29, 179–183

158. .Dobrovolskaia-Zavadskaia, N. (1927) Sur la mortification spontanee de la queue chez la souris nouveax-nee et sur l'existence d'un caractere heriditaire 'non-viable'. C.R. Soc. Biol., 97, 114–116.

159. .Wilkinson, D.G., Bhatt, S. and Herrmann, B.G. (1990) Expression pattern of the mouse *T* gene and its role in mesoderm formation. Nature, 343, 567–659.

160. .Bamshad, M., Lin, R.C., Law, D.J., Watkins, W.S., Krakowiak, P.A., Moore, M.E., Franceschini, B., Lala, R., Holmes, L.B., Gebuhr, T.C. *et al.* (1997) Mutations in human *TBX3* alter limb, apocrine and genital development in ulnar-mammary syndrome. Nat. Genet., 16, 311–315.

161. .Basson, C.T., Backinscky, D.R., Lin, R.C., Levi, T., Elkins, J.A., Soults, J., Grayzel, D., Kroumpousou, K., Trail, T.A., Leblanc-Straceski, J. *et al.* (1997) Mutations in human *TBX5* cause limb and cardiac malformations in Holt–Oram syndrome. Nat. Genet., 15, 30–35.

162. .Jerome, L.A. and Papaioannou, V.E. (2001) DiGeorge syndrome phenotype in mice mutant for the T-box gene, Tbx1. Nat. Genet., 27, 286–291.

163. .Lindsey, E.A., Vitelli, F., Su, H., Morishima, M., Huynh, T., Pramparo, T., Jurecic, V., Ogunrinu, G., Sutherland, H.F., Scambler, P.J. *et al.* (2001) *Tbx1*haploinsufficiency in the DiGeorge syndrome region causes aortic arch defects in mice. Nature, 410, 97–101.

164. .Lamolet, B., Pulichino, A.M., Lamonerie, T., Gauthier, Y., Brue, T., Enjalbert, A. and Drouin, J. (2001) A pituitary cell-restricted T box factor, Tpit, activates POMC transcription in cooperation with Pitx homeoproteins. Cell, 104, 849–859.

165. .Marçano, A.C.B., Doudney, K., Braybrook, C., Squires, R., Patton, M.A., Lees, M., Richieri-Costa, A., Lideral, A.C., Murray, J.C., Moore, G.E. and Stanier, P. (2004)*TBX22* mutations are a frequent cause of cleft palate. J. Med. Genet., 41, 68–74.

166. .Gorski, S.M., Adams, K.J., Birch, P.H., Chodirker, B.N., Greenberg, C.R. and Goodfellow, P.J. (1994) Linkage analysis of X-linked cleft palate and ankyloglossia in Manitoba Menonite and British Columbia Native kindreds Hum. Genet., 94, 141–148.

167. .Basson, C.T., Huang, T., Lin, R.C., Bachinsky, D.R., Weremowicz, S., Vaglio, A., Bruzzone, R., Quadrelli, R., Lerone, M., Romeo, G. *et al.* (1999) Different *TBX5*interactions in heart and limb defined by Holt-Oram syndrome mutations. Proc. Natl Acad. Sci. USA, 96, 2919–2924.

168. .Ghosh, T.K., Packham, E.A., Bonser, A.J., Robinson, T.E., Cross, S.J. and Brook, J.D. (2001) Characterization of the *TBX5* binding site and analysis of mutations that cause Holt–Oram syndrome. Hum. Mol. Genet., 10, 1983–1994.

169. .Fan, C., Liu, M. and Wang, Q. (2003) Functional analysis of TBX5 missense mutations associated with holt-oram syndrome. J. Biol. Chem., 278, 8780–8785.

170. .Braybrook, C., Lisgo, S., Doudney, K., Henderson, D., Marçano, A.C.B., Strachan, T., Patton, M.A., Villard, L., Moore, G.E., Stanier, P. and

Lindsay, S. (2002) Craniofacial expression of human and murine *TBX22* correlates with the cleft palate and ankyloglossia phenotype observed in CPX patients. Hum. Mol. Genet., 11,2793–2804.

171. .Bush, J.O., Lan, Y., Maltby, K.M. and Jiang, R. (2002) Isolation and developmental expression analysis of *Tbx22*, the mouse homolog of the human X-linked cleft palate gene. Dev. Dyn., 225, 322–326.

172. .Haenig, B., Schmidt, C., Kraus, F., Pfordt, M. and Kispert, A. (2002) Cloning and expression analysis of the chick ortholog of *TBX22*, the gene mutated in X-linked cleft palate and ankyloglossia. Mech. Dev., 117, 321–325.

173. .Suzuki, K., Hu, D., Bustos, T., Zlotogora, J., Richieri-Costa, A., Helms, J.A. and Spritz, R.A. (2000) Mutations of *PVRL1*, encoding a cell-cell adhesion molecule/herpesvirus receptor, in cleft lip/palate-ectodermal dysplasia. Nat. Genet., 25, 427–430.

174. .Suzuki, K., Hu, D., Bustos, T., Zlotogora, J., Richieri-Costa, A., Helms, J.A. and Spritz, R.A. (2000) Mutations of PVRL1, encoding a cell-cell adhesion molecule/herpesvirus receptor, in cleft lip/palate-ectodermal dysplasia. Nat. Genet., 25, 427–430.

175. .Geraghty, R.J., Krummenacher, C., Cohen, G.H., Eisenberg, R.J. and Spear, P.G. (1998) Entry of alphaherpesviruses mediated by poliovirus receptor-related protein 1 and poliovirus receptor. Science, 280, 1618–1620.

176. .Sozen, M.A., Suzuki, K., Talavora, M.M., Bustos, T., Fernandez Iglesias, J.E. and Spritz, R.A. (2001) Mutation of *PVRL1* is associated with sporadic, non-syndromic cleft lip/palate in northern Venezuela. Nat. Genet., 29, 141–142.

177. .Kondo, S., Schutte, B.C., Richardson, R.J., Bjork, B.C., Knight, A.S., Watanabe, Y., Howard, E., de Lima, R.L., Daack-Hirsch, S., Sander, A. *et al.* (2002) Mutations in *IRF6* cause Van der Woude and popliteal pterygium syndromes. Nat. Genet., 32,285–289.

178. .Zucchero, T., Cooper, M., Caprau, D., Ribero, L., Suzuki, Y., Yoshiura, K., Christiensen, K., Moreno, L., Johnson, M., Field, L. *et al.* (2003) *IRF6* is a major modifier for nonsyndromic cleft with or without cleft palate. Am. J. Hum. Genet., 73,A4.

179. .Prescott, N., Garcia-Rodriguez, C., Lees, M. and Winter, R.M. (2003) Candidate genes in nonsyndromic cleft lip and palate. Am. J. Hum. Genet., 73, A727.

180. .Celli, J., Duijf, P., Hamel, B.C., Bamshad, M., Kramer, B., Smits, A.P., Newbury-Ecob, R., Hennekam, R.C., Van Buggenhout, G., van Haeringen, A. *et al.* (1999) Heterozygous germline mutations in the p53 homolog p63 are the cause of EEC syndrome. Cell, 99, 143–153.

181. ...Barrow, L.L., van Bokhoven, H., Daack-Hirsch, S., Andersen, T., van Beersum, S.E., Gorlin, R. and Murray, J.C. (2002) Analysis of the p63 gene in classical EEC syndrome, related syndromes, and non-syndromic orofacial clefts. J. Med. Genet.,39, 559–566.

182. 183.Jiang, R., Lan, Y., Chapman, H.D., Shawber, C., Norton, C.R., Serreze, D.V., Weinmaster, G. and Gridley, T. Defects in limb, craniofacial, and thymic development in Jagged2 mutant mice. Genes Dev., 12, 1046–1057.

183. .Lidral, A.C., Romitti, P.A., Basart, A.M., Doetschman, T., Leysens, N.J., Daack-Hirsch, S., Semina, E.V., Johnson, L.R., Machida, J., Burds, A. *et al.* (1998) Association of MSX1 and TGFB3 with nonsyndromic clefting in humans. Am. J. Hum. Genet., 63, 557–568.

184. .Van den Boogard, M.-J.H., Dorland, M., Beemer, F.A. and Ploos van Amstel, H.K. (2000) *MSX1* mutation is associated with orofacial clefting and tooth agenesis in humans. Nat. Genet., 24, 342–343.

185. .Hecht, J.T., Mulliken, J.B. and Blanton, S.H. (2002) Evidence for a cleft palate only locus on chromosome 4 near MSX1. Am. J. Med. Genet., 110, 406–407.

186. .Vieira, A.R., Orioli, I.M., Castilla, E.E., Cooper, M.E., Marazita, M.L. and Murray, J.C. (2003) *MSX1* and *TGFB3* contribute to clefting in South America. J. Dent. Res., 82,289–292.

187. .Jugessur, A., Lie, R.T., Wilcox, A.J., Murray, J.C., Taylor, J.A., Saugstad, O.D., Vindenes, H.A. and Abyholm, F. (2003) Variants of developmental genes (*TGFA, TGFB3,* and *MSX1*) and their associations with orofacial clefts: a case-parent triad analysis. Genet.Epidemiol., 24, 230–239.

188. .Fallin, M.D., Hetmanski, J.B., Park, J., Scott, A.F., Ingersoll, R., Fuernkranz, H.A., McIntosh, I. and Beaty, T.H. (2003) Family-based analysis of MSX1 haplotypes for association with oral clefts. Genet.Epidemiol., 25, 168–17

189. 190.Mitchell, L.E., Murray, J.C., O'Brien, S. and Christensen, K. (2001) Evaluation of two putative susceptibility loci for oral clefts in the Danish population. Am. J. Epidemiol., 153, 1007–1015.

190. .Koillinen, H., Ollikainen, V., Rautio, J., Hukki, J. and Kere, J. (2003) Linkage and linkage disequilibrium searched for between non-syndromic cleft palate and four candidate loci. J. Med. Genet., 40, 464–468.

191. .Jezewski, P., Vieira, A., Schultz, R., Machida, J., Suzuki, Y., Ludwig, B., Daack-Hirsch, S., O'Brian, S., Nishimura, C., Johnson, M. and Murray, J.C. (2003) Mutations in *MSX1* are associated with non-syndromic orofacial clefting. J. Med. Genet., 40,399–407.

192. .Dode, C., Levilliers, J., Dupont, J.M., De Paepe, A., Le Du, N., Soussi-Yanicostas, N., Coimbra, R.S., Delmaghani, S., Compain-Nouaille, S.,

Baverel, F. *et al.* (2003) Loss-of-function mutations in *FGFR1* cause autosomal dominant Kallmann syndrome. Nat. Genet., 33, 463–465.

193. .Clifton-Bligh, R.J., Wentworth, J.M., Heinz, P., Crisp, M.S., John, R., Lazarus, J.H., Ludgate, M. and Chatterjee, V.K. (1998) Mutation of the gene encoding human *TTF-2* associated with thyroid agenesis, cleft palate and choanal atresia. Nat. Genet.,19, 399–401.

194. .Fang, J., Dagenais, S.L., Erickson, R.P., Arlt, M.F., Glynn, M.W., Gorski, J.L., Seaver, L.H. and Glover, T.W. (2000) Mutations in *FOXC2* (MFH-1), a forkhead family transcription factor, are responsible for the hereditary lymphedema–distichiasis syndrome. Am. J. Hum. Genet., 67, 1382–1388.

195. .FitzPatrick, D.R., Carr, I.M., McLaren, L., Leek, J.P., Wightman, P., Williamson, K., Gautier, P., McGill, N., Hayward, C., Firth, H. *et al.* (2003) Identification of *SATB2* as the cleft palate gene on 2q32-q33. Hum. Mol. Genet., 12, 2491–2501.

196. .Beiraghi, S., Zhou, M. Talmadge, C.B., Went-Sumegi, N., Davis, J.R., Huang, D., Saal, H., Seemayer, T.A. and Sumegi, J. (2003) Identification and characterization of a novel gene disrupted by a pericentric inversion inv(4)(p13.1q21.1) in a family with cleft lip. Gene, 309, 11–21.

197. .Brown, N.L., Knott, L., Halligan, E., Yarram, S.J., Mansell, J.P. and Sandy, J.R. (2003) Microarray analysis of murine palatogenesis: Temporal expression of genes during normal palate development. Dev. Growth Differ., 45, 153–165.

198. .Fowles, L.F., Bennetts, J.S., Berkman, J.L., Williams, E., Koopman, P., Teasdale, R.D. and Wicking, C. (2003) Genomic screen for genes involved in mammalian craniofacial development. Genesis, 35, 73–87.

199. .Adams D.A.the exauset of deafness .In scott Byowr's Otolarynyology 5th ed. Edited by KerrA.G.London Butterworth 1987;6;35

200. .Hechet JT et al non syndromic cleft lip and palate noi evidence of linkage to IILA or factor 13 A AM J HUN Genet !((#; 52 F6 ;1230

201. Johnson MC Hassel JR, Brown K.S.the embryology of cleft lip and palate clinic plastic surgery 1975;2;195

202. Terry P.B. Bissenden JG condic R.J. Methew P.M Ethenic Differences In congenital malformation Arch Dischild 1985 ;60;865

203. .Salder TW congenital malformation .In Langma's Medical embryology 5th ed. Edited by tracy T.M. Baltimore Williams And Wilkins 1985 ; 102

204. Shupback PM experimental induction of an incomplete hard palate cleft in the rat. Oral sug.oral med oral path 1983 ;55,2

205. .Pashley NRT Kruse CJ ,cleft lip cleft palate and other fusion disorders .The Otolaryngol clinic North 1981;14 ;125

206. .Jons Kl ,Environmental agent fetal aminoprotein effects .In smith's recognizable pattern of human malformation 4th ed. Edited by jons V.L. Philadeilhia W.B. Saunders company 1988;506

207. .Allen RW et al Fetal hydontion syndrome ;neuroblastoma and hemmorrrhagic diseases in neonates JAMA , 1980 ;244:1464

208. .Maniglia AJ ,Embryology Teratology and arrested developmental disorder in otolaryngology .The otolaryngol clinic north America 1981;14;25

209. nemana BJ Marazita MC Menick M > genetic analysis of cleft lip withot cleft palate in Madras America Journal med general 1992 ; 42 (1) 5; 9

210. Rintala A. Reneta R . Stegars T. on the pathogenesis of cleft palate in pierre robin syndrome Scand J Plastic reconstruction surgery 1984 ; 18; 37 inc 1983;13

211. young malformation in different ethenic groupsw Arch Dis child !987 ;62;103

212. Gooday RHB ,precious DS duplication of mental nerve in patient with a cleft lip palate and Rubell syndrome .Oral sug. Med .med oral pathology 1988 ;65 : 157

213. Clarren SK ,smithy DW ,The fetal alcohol syndrome N English journal med. 1978 jan 29 (1) 15-6

214. .Davis JS and H.P Richie classification of congenital clefts of lip and the palate JAMA 79,16,1323-1332 , 1992

215. .kernhan D.A.Stark R.B.A new classification of cleft lip and palate Reconstructive surgery 1958:22:435-445

216. Tessier, P., "Anatomical Classification of Facial, Cranio-Facial and Latero-Facial Clefts" Journalof Maxillofacial Surgery, 1976 4 (69-92)

217. .Converse, chapter 38:John Marquis Converse,V.Michel Hogan , Joshph,G. Mccarthy.

218. .converse ,chapter 43:the unilateral cleft lip by:Ross H.Musgrave ,William S,Garrenett ,JR

219. .Rose W. on hair lip and palate 1891

220. .Thompson JE . An artistic and mathematically accurate method of repairing of defect in case of haire lip .surgery Gyneal obstat 1921 ; 14 ;498 -504

221. .Analysis and evolution of rotation principles inunilateral cleft lip repairJoshua C. Demke a,*, Sherard A. Tatum b

   a. Facial Plastic and Reconstructive Surgery Division of Otolaryngology, Department of Surgery, Texas Tech University,School of Medicine, 3601 4th Street, Lubbock, TX 79430, USA

   b. Division of Facial Plastic and Reconstructive Surgery, SUNY Upstate Medical University, Syracuse, NY, USA Received 9 November 2009; accepted 1 March 2010

222. .The roatation –advancement technique (Millard) as asecondary procedure in cleft lip deformities by:Saul Hoffman M.D., David R. Wesser M.D.Fanny Calostypis M.D. Bernard E Simon M.D.

223. Delaire J. :Theoretical principles and technique of funbctional closure of lip and nasal aperture j. maxillofacial surgery 1978: 6: 1:1996

224. . Text book of pedodontics by: shobha tandon.

225. .Division OF Plastic recotruction and cosmatic surgery .The university of ILLIMOS at chicago,958820,south wood street cook country chicago,II 60612,USA

226. .clinics in palatine surgery (2004)331-345 resudual defomities after repaire of cleft lip anad palate Mimis Cohen ,M.D,.FACS,FAA.

227. .STAL. S.Hollier C. Coorection of secondary cleft lip deformities plastic recontructive surgery 2002,109:1677-1681.

228. .Millard JR DR shaping and positing the lip ,switch flap in unilateral cleft,InMillard JR DR editor ,cleft craft evaolution of its surgery vol-I Boston little brown and co. 1976 PS 93 -628

229. .Late correction of orbicularies discontinuty of bilateral cleft defomity.Vharles C.PUCKETT ,M.D. FACS JOHN F REINISH,M.D. RICHER S. WERNE M.D. COLOMBIA,MISSOURI 65212

230. Kawamoto Jr HK.Correction of major defects of vermilion with a cross-lip vermilion flap. Plast Rec Surg 1974;64:315– 8.

231. Hogan VH, Converse JM. Secondary deformities of unilateral cleft lip and nose. In: Grabb WC, Rosenstein SC, Bzoch KR, editors. Cleft lip and palate: surgical, dental and speech aspects. Boston: Little, Brown and Co.; 1971.p. 245– 61.

232. Kapetansky D. Double pendulum flaps for whistling deformities in bilateral cleft lip.Plast Rec Surg 1971; 47:321–3. [12] Rodgers CH,

233. Emory RE, Clay RP, Bite U, Jackson I. Fistula formationand repair after palatal closure: an institutionalperspective. Plast Rec Surg 1997;99:1535– 8.

234. . Cohen M, Smith BE, Daw J. Secondary unilateral cleftlip nasal deformity: functional and aesthetic reconstruction.J Craniofacial Surg 2003;14:584– 93.

235. . Cohen M. Secondary correction of the nasal deformity associated with cleft lip. In: Cohen M, editor. Mastery of plastic and reconstructive surgery, vol. 1. Boston: Little, Brown and Company; 1994. p. 702– 19.

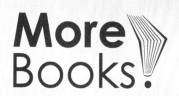
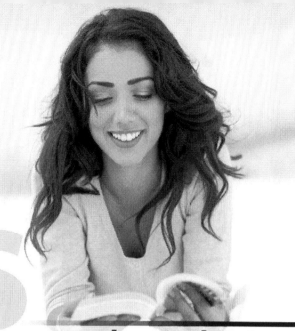

Printed in Great Britain
by Amazon

75897886R00122